Addressing Challenging Moments in Psychotherapy

‖‖‖‖‖‖‖‖‖‖‖‖‖‖
W0113496

This practical and helpful volume details how clinicians can work through various common challenges in individual, couple, or group psychotherapy.

Chapters draw upon clinical wisdom gleaned from the author's 48 years as a practicing psychiatrist to address topics such as using countertransference for therapeutic purposes; resistance, especially when it needs to be the focus of the therapy; and a prioritization of exploration over explanation. Along with theory and clinical observations, Dr Gans offers a series of "Clinical Pearls," pithy comments that highlight different interventions to a wide range of clinical challenges. These include patient hostility, the abrupt and unilateral termination of therapy, the therapist's loss of compassionate neutrality when treating a couple, and many more. Many of the "Clinical Pearls" prioritize working in the here-and-now. In addition to offering advice and strategies for therapists, the book also addresses concerns like the matter of fees in private practice and the virtue of moral courage on the part of the therapist.

Written with clarity, heart, and an abundance of clinical wisdom, *Addressing Challenging Moments in Psychotherapy* is essential reading for all clinicians, teachers, and supervisors of psychotherapy.

Jerome S. Gans, MD, is a Distinguished Life Fellow of the American Group Psychotherapy Association and the American Psychiatric Association. Now retired, he previously worked in private practice and as Associate Clinical Professor of Psychiatry, Harvard Medical School.

The New International Library of Group Analysis (NILGA)
Series Editor: Earl Hopper

Drawing on the seminal ideas of British, European and American group analysts, psychoanalysts, social psychologists and social scientists, the books in this series focus on the study of small and large groups, organizations and other social systems, and on the study of the transpersonal and transgenerational sociality of human nature. NILGA books will be required reading for the members of professional organizations in the field of group analysis, psychoanalysis, and related social sciences. They will be indispensable for the "formation" of students of psychotherapy, whether they are mainly interested in clinical work with patients or in consultancy to teams and organizational clients within the private and public sectors.

Recent titles in the series include:

The Portuguese School of Group Analysis
Towards a Unified and Integrated Approach to Theory Research and Clinical Work
Edited by Isaura Manso Neto and Margarida França

Richard M. Billow's Selected Papers on Psychoanalysis and Group Process
Changing Our Minds
Edited by Tzachi Slonim

Addressing Challenging Moments in Psychotherapy
Clinical Wisdom for Working with Individuals, Groups and Couples
Jerome S. Gans

Psychoanalysis, Group Analysis, and Beyond
Towards a New Paradigm of the Human Being
Juan Tubert-Oklander and Reyna Hernández-Tubert

For more information about this series, please visit: www.routledge.com/The-New-International-Library-of-Group-Analysis/book-series/KARNNILGA

"This book is the wonderfully rich distillation of 48 years of experience treating individuals, couples and groups in a variety of settings. Dr Gans shows his considerable wisdom and compassion throughout the variety of clinical examples. He covers a wide variety of therapeutic challenges ranging from threatened suicide to seemingly casual remarks. The book offers a compelling combination of thoughtful and sophisticated analysis with eminently clear writing and will help clinicians at all levels to reflect more deeply about each therapy session they conduct."

Eleanor F. Counselman, EdD, ABPP, CGP, DLFAGPA,
Distinguished Fellow and immediate past President,
the American Group Psychotherapy Association

"Dr. Gans writes with clarity and deep appreciation for the psychotherapeutic process. His book illuminates the ways in which effective therapists must use themselves expertly as therapeutic agents, fully integrating their knowledge, understanding, compassion and humanity. Throughout, he demonstrates how the values of therapist decency and deep care for our patients, interface with our theories and techniques. Gans writes with passion, wisdom, humor and abiding respect for his patients and their inspiring courage and resilience."

Molyn Leszcz, MD, FRCPC, CGP, DFAGPA,
Professor of Psychiatry, University of Toronto
and President, the American Group
Psychotherapy Association

"It is a cause for celebration when a highly experienced, trusted clinician and teacher, such as Jerry Gans, delivers a work that is as fresh, original, stimulating, provocative and *helpful* as this book. It reflects a current wish for more creative and innovative ways of working and offers numerous valuable ideas for interacting with clients in unconventional but impactful ways, in individual, couple and group therapy. Paradox, irony and surprise abound. The author offers not just his own ideas but encourages readers to find their own voice as psychotherapists: free, spontaneous and playful."

Morris Nitsun, *Training Analyst, the Institute of Group*
Analysis, London, and author of The Anti-Group *and*
The Group as an Object of Desire

"In his book, Dr. Gans weaves selected clinical pearls. Shame, marital discord, countertransferance and pain—Gans illuminates different aspects related to relationships. Skillfully and lovingly he leads us to the depth of the challenge inherent in the therapeutic encounter. With characteristic eloquence and sincerity, he captures the reader's heart as he shares interventions, explains rationale and shares powerful insights."

Sharon Sagi Berg, MA, *Group Analyst, Psychotherapist,*
Director of Tel Aviv Schema Therapy Center

Addressing Challenging Moments in Psychotherapy

Clinical Wisdom for Working with Individuals, Groups and Couples

Jerome S. Gans

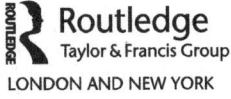
Routledge
Taylor & Francis Group

LONDON AND NEW YORK

First published 2022
by Routledge
2 Park Square, Milton Park, Abingdon, Oxon OX14 4RN

and by Routledge
605 Third Avenue, New York, NY 10158

Routledge is an imprint of the Taylor & Francis Group, an informa business

© 2022 Jerome S. Gans

The right of Jerome S. Gans to be identified as author of this
work has been asserted by him in accordance with sections 77
and 78 of the Copyright, Designs and Patents Act 1988.

All rights reserved. No part of this book may be reprinted
or reproduced or utilized in any form or by any electronic,
mechanical, or other means, now known or hereafter invented,
including photocopying and recording, or in any information
storage or retrieval system, without permission in writing from
the publishers.

Trademark notice: Product or corporate names may be trademarks
or registered trademarks, and are used only for identification and
explanation without intent to infringe.

British Library Cataloguing-in-Publication Data
A catalogue record for this book is available from the British Library

Library of Congress Cataloging-in-Publication Data
A catalog record for this book has been requested

ISBN: 978-1-032-00533-1 (hbk)
ISBN: 978-1-032-00532-4 (pbk)
ISBN: 978-1-003-17460-8 (ebk)

DOI: 10.4324/9781003174608

Typeset in Times New Roman
by Apex CoVantage, LLC

To my wife Nancy,
the love of my life and my very best editor.

Tell all the Truth but tell it slant –
Success in Circuit lies
Too bright for our infirm Delight
To Truth's superb surprise

As lightning to the Children eased
With explanation kind
The Truth must dazzle gradually
Or every man be blind.

Emily Dickinson, in *Dickinson:
Selected Poems and
Commentaries Helen Vendler*,
p. 431 (Cambridge, MA:
The Belnap Press of
Harvard University
Press, 2010)

"Doc, it's amazing to me the things you sometimes have to say to your patients to help them."

Said to me by a group patient

Contents

Foreword

When starting to write this Foreword to such a personal and perhaps unique contribution to the theoretically informed clinical practice of group psychotherapy by Jerome Gans, MD, the first words that came to my mind were personal, intimate, honest, courageous, wise, and ironically humorous. Dr Gans writes from a relational space that is characterized by an ethical commitment to be true to his self in the service of guiding his patients and students in the exploration of their personalities, identities, and relationships that are not yet fully known to them. We are invited to collect his clinical pearls slowly, one by one, until they are apperceived into a new object, something like a bracelet or a necklace of emblematic jewelry. Like a Catholic rosary or a Greek komboloi, Jerry's transitional objects of experience and hope help us both to understand and to manage our witching hours. His Book of Recollections of moments of meeting in individual, group, and couple psychotherapy is saturated with warmth and feeling. That life is hallmarked by the challenge to transform grit into natural pearls, no one of which is identical to another, is at the heart of our being able to learn from experience, and especially of being able to make creative use of traumatic experience.

If he were a member of the group analytic and psychoanalytic communities in Britain, Dr Gans would almost certainly be an independent who takes his inspiration from both Freud and Klein, and from both Foulkes and Bion. He would be associated with the traditions of Winnicott, Millner, and Rycroft and in general with those of us who most deeply appreciate the sociality of human nature and the complexities of the socially unconscious dimensions of it. I very much appreciate the contributions and personal styles of those by whom Jerry has been mentored. He fully expresses his gratitude toward a diverse selection of guides and teachers in a professional field which is so often a wilderness, if not a dangerous warzone. In turn, we are offered an opportunity to be mentored vicariously.

Although deeply informed by developments in psychoanalytical and group analytical theory, Jerry is guided by what "works." I look forward to using this book for teaching both new and more advanced students. My colleagues will also benefit from and enjoy the ideas that are so beautifully explicated in this aesthetically and intellectually satisfying book by one of the contemporary fathers of group psychotherapy in the United States, especially in the Boston area, where he has had a long and distinguished career as a therapist, teacher, and professional colleague. I am very pleased to be able to introduce him to group analysts in Britain and in Europe more generally.

Earl Hopper, PhD
Series Editor

Acknowledgments

My mentors, teachers, and influential colleagues have been men and women psychiatrists, psychologists, teachers, and coaches (listed in the order in which they influenced me personally and professionally): Ray Iman, Mauro Panaggio, Charles Whitlock, John Romano, George Engel, Elvin Semrad, Jack Ewalt, Elizabeth Zetzel, Lenore Boling, Leston Havens, Max Day, Dan Asnes, Bernard Lown, Thomas Gutheil, Anne Alonso, Scott Rutan, Eleanor Counselman, Libby Shapiro, Richard Billow, and Adam Silk. Rabbi Harold Kushner helped me to appreciate what is important in life. For 30 years, I have been in peer supervision with Arnie Cohen, Suzanne Cohen, Steve Krugman, and Geri Reinhardt. Many of my ideas have evolved in conversations with them.

My wife, Nancy, read and made helpful comments on every draft of the book. I learned in writing this book that if Nancy didn't understand parts of it, I wasn't being clear. Her focus and clarity of thinking can be found in every chapter. Her support throughout the writing of this book has been unflagging.

For reading and commenting on parts of the manuscript, many thanks to Chap Attwell, Mark Bauer, Arnie Cohen, Suzanne Cohen, Eleanor Counselman, Bob Ferrell, David Fine, Dale Godby, Earl Hopper, Bob Klein, Dan Leinweber, Scott Rutan, and Libby Shapiro. Thanks for comments from a group of Chinese therapists I've been teaching and learning from on Zoom, using chapters of this book. They are Shuai Li, Fang Zhang, Hao Yu, Wang Bei, Yang Hui, Li Lu, Zhong Shen, Wang Yongfen, Li Chunman, and Sarah Wu. Yang Lihua's superb simultaneous translating greatly facilitated my teaching. I'm indebted to Richard Lansing for his superb editing of the entire book. David Fine brought Emily Dickinson's poem to my attention. Jeffrey Roth and Elaine Cooper read the entire manuscript and offered helpful suggestions. I'm indebted to my friend, colleague, and artist, David Altfeld, whose painting appears on the cover of my book.

Part 1

Introduction

Introduction

In my 48 years as a practicing psychiatrist, I have listened to approximately 80,000 hours of patients' stories and supervised approximately 90 psychotherapists. I have worked in a variety of settings. These include working as a liaison psychiatrist in both a cardiac care unit and in an acute physical rehabilitation hospital. I have worked as a staff psychiatrist in a mental hospital and run T-groups (training groups) for two major psychiatric residency programs. Over that period of time, I had either a part-time or full-time private psychotherapy practice treating individuals, couples, and running psychotherapy groups.

This book is a collection of clinical observations and aphorisms that I have culled from my experience treating patients and supervising therapists. The book gives examples of the wonderful variety of challenging moments in psychotherapy. Here are a few.

- A patient introduces himself by telling you in an intimidating manner that the magazines in your waiting room are out of date—and that he wants current ones when he returns next week.
- You realize to your dismay that you've been exploiting the diplomatic nature of one of your group members to calm group conflict.
- You wonder how you will be able gradually to nudge a chronic complainer into self-reflection.
- You find yourself consistently very sleepy three-quarters of the way through a session when you were wide awake at the beginning of the session.
- You notice that your patient's excessive vagueness is turning your brain into cotton candy.
- You look at your appointment book and realize you are dreading the next therapy hour because it is with Marvin.
- An unhappily married woman convincingly explains to you in individual therapy that her husband was "never like that" before she married him.
- Your group patient tells you that your answering her question with a question feels disrespectful and causes her to shut down.
- You feel anxious when with 5 minutes left in the session your patient mentions that she is feeling suicidal.

DOI: 10.4324/9781003174608-2

- Your decision not to look at your patient and instead "talk to the room" is advancing the therapy.
- Your supervisee asks for your help in dealing with a question her patient just asked her, "What do you think of me?"
- Your long-term patient who has done very well in a 5-year therapy invites you and your spouse to her wedding.

The first part of this book highlights clinical observations I've made about human nature taken from the various settings in which I have worked as a psychiatrist. These observations serve as background and inform my responses to challenging moments in psychotherapy that I discuss in the second part of the book. Over the years I have learned that in most instances people are doing the best they can; meaningful therapeutic work takes place at the boundaries; there is much that we can learn about ourselves from our patients; and many natural reactions are not helpful and many helpful reactions do not come naturally. I welcome these challenges as an expected part of the ongoing psychotherapeutic work.

In the second part of the book, I put these challenging moments in long-term psychotherapy under a magnifying glass. I describe my interventions to these challenging moments and refer to them as Clinical Pearls. The term refers to pithy comments I have made to my patients and my supervisees in the service of advancing the therapy. The Clinical Pearls confront complexity and make it appear deceptively simple. I then unpack these Clinical Pearls by explaining the thinking that went into their construction, articulation, and goals. The Clinical Pearls condense what I have learned in the course of working with two major groups of individuals: my patients and my supervisees.

A few years ago, I decided to make a list of these Clinical Pearls after many of my patients and supervisees said that I have a of way of concisely sharing clinical insights that they have found helpful both professionally and personally. For example, neophyte therapists who were my supervisees felt understood—given their financial struggles—when I suggested that the best supervisor is a mortgage. (If I had 1200 words to say about that remark, I would have made it a Clinical Pearl.) At the time I didn't have the energy or the time to expand on the thinking that went into these aphorisms. Now, largely confined to my home during the pandemic, I have time to spare and, with my retirement over a year ago, renewed energy. While writing about the Clinical Pearls, I have been mindful of a medical school teaching about clinical pearls: they are the same size as rabbit turds. You, my readers, will make that determination as you read on.

I would characterize my general approach to patients as indirect. Drawing on my undergraduate experience as a major in English literature, I employ in my interventions with clients a wide number of literary devices such as irony, paradox, exaggeration, indirection, surprise, and humor. The Clinical Pearls attempt to achieve a variety of goals. In the various clinical examples provided, they secure attention, promote safety, respect choice, and foster a sense of agency. By conveying empathy, they serve to deepen affect, welcome transference, and replace grim antagonism with playful curiosity. They prioritize exploration over explanation and embrace complexity. They employ countertransference for therapeutic purposes. Cognitively, the Clinical Pearls help clarify communication and promote consolidation and integration of discoveries.

The Clinical Pearls address many clinical topics. They educate patients about basic rules of psychotherapy, monitor the therapeutic alliance, and offer guidance in dealing with patients' questions. In addressing character pathology, they strive to make the ego-syntonic dystonic. In processing transference and countertransference, they deepen affect, especially negative feelings. They assist the therapist in treating the suicidal patient and other self-destructive conditions. They encourage and give value and appeal to imagination, authenticity, creativity, and spontaneity.

I have disguised case material taken from my private practice and from my supervisees' practices. My patients have come from across all sectors of the socioeconomic spectrum. The patients range from their early 20s to their late 80s. Early in my career, I treated psychotic patients as well as the neurotic, character-disordered, depressed, anxious, and bereaved patients who comprised my patient roster as time went on. While I have treated many patients with adjustment disorders, I have not included examples from this population in the book. The reason for this omission is that the book deals more with patients' internal worlds and persistent conflicts than with temporary external problems.

The material in this book, for the most part, has resisted neat categorization. Some of the clinical examples can be grouped under the headings of individual, group, and couple therapy. Over half of the Clinical Pearls deal with the patient–therapist relationship primarily in the here-and-now. The many clinical examples discuss the use of countertransference for therapeutic purposes. The Clinical Pearls seek to advance the therapy by promoting self-reflection, strengthening the therapeutic alliance, favoring exploration over explanation, and fostering curiosity and stimulating imagination. The first 11 chapters contain insights about human nature that I have encountered in the therapy hour. The next ten chapters each contain two Clinical Pearls except for the chapter on using countertransference for clinical purposes that contains four Clinical Pearls and the miscellaneous chapter that contains three Clinical Pearls.

One more comment about the last ten chapters. In earlier drafts, each of the 22 Clinical Pearls was one chapter. For smoother reading, I condensed the 22 chapters into 10. This was a complicated task because each Clinical Pearl mentions and illustrates a number of psychotherapy-related topics. My task in forming each of these ten chapters was to select two Clinical Pearls (and four in the chapter on countertransference) appropriate to each chapter heading—even though the Clinical Pearls originally were not written with those chapter headings in mind. Again, you the reader, will decide the success of these pairings. The perfect is the enemy of the good.

I want to offer a cautionary note especially to younger readers about the use of Clinical Pearls that comes from my early clinical training. During my psychiatric residency, I had the privilege of observing the work of Dr Elvin Semrad, a wonderful teacher of psychotherapy at the Massachusetts Mental Health Center in Boston. At case conferences he would interview patients we had been working with for months. He had an uncanny way of relating to very sick patients by using simple language to address profound suffering. For example, he would say to the patient, "Tell me, what is breaking your heart?" and, before we knew it, the patient was divulging material that we hadn't unearthed in months of sitting with the patient. We residents were so impressed with Dr Semrad's seemingly magical ability to have patients reveal their innermost thoughts and feelings that we immediately left the case conference and asked our next patient, "So tell me, what is breaking your heart?" Of course, in our hands, that approach fell flat. And how could it not have, since that intervention did not come from our authentic experience and sense of self. So, consider the Clinical Pearls as only one approach to a challenging moment in psychotherapy. Find your way to approach such a challenging moment that fits you and your way of doing therapy with a particular patient. Find the uniqueness of every patient and select from all the approaches those that have the greatest chance of improving the treatment. If my thinking discussed in the formulation and use of the Clinical Pearl contributes to your therapeutic personhood, I will be more than pleased. Continue evolving your distinctive therapeutic presence.

Who is the audience for this book? This book will interest therapists who treat patients in long-term individual, group, or couples psychotherapy. Both clinical practitioners and educators/trainers will find the book useful because it deals with clinical situations that both neophyte and seasoned clinicians struggle with. It will appeal to those who welcome the dark sides of human nature into their offices. The book will engage therapists who use their countertransference for therapeutic purposes, especially those attentive to the possibility that they might be impeding the very therapeutic enterprise they are trying to promote. The Clinical Pearls will provide interesting clinical material for those who wish to expand their use of innovative therapeutic techniques that involve spontaneity, playfulness, and creativity. Several chapters address moments in therapy especially challenging for neophyte therapists. Older clinicians—I am now 80—will resonate with the emphasis on compassion, kindness, and respect for the patient. Therapists in the middle years of their careers might find approaches to complement or possibly challenge their current practice. The clinical observations and Clinical Pearls may provide additional tools to supervisors of psychotherapy. Also, for those considering entering into psychotherapy training, the book might serve as an additional inducement to explore their concerns. Because I evolved some of the ideas in this book while working as a liaison psychiatrist in both a cardiac unit and an acute physical rehabilitation hospital, the book may prove useful to mental health professionals who work with physical therapists, occupational therapists, speech therapists, and nurses—and, perhaps, physicians interested in the psychological aspects of patient care.

For as long as I can remember, I have taken delight in the diversity of human nature. It is no wonder then that as a psychotherapist I have embraced a pluralistic approach to the work. I have tried in my career to put into practice the statement of the Roman playwright and poet Terrence, who said "Homo sum; humani nil a me alienum puto," "I am a man (person); I think nothing human is alien (foreign) to me." I hope that readers find that this book enhances the treatment of their patients and brings new life to their clinical practices.

Part II

Clinical observations

Chapter 1

There are no completely objective data in interpersonal relations. The way I am with you partly determines the way you are with me.

It is impressive how many years it took the field of psychotherapy/psychoanalysis to appreciate that the classic definition of transference was limited. The original idea of transference was that if the analyst was interested, reliable, curious, impassive, and non-judgmental, over time the patient would begin to experience the analyst as an important person from the patient's past with whom the patient experienced unresolved conflict. The patient would begin to relate to the analyst as if he or she were that important person from the patient's past. Only this time, because the analyst was not in reality that person and because the analyst was devoted to helping the patient resolve these conflicts, the patient's transference could be analyzed and the patient freed up from his/her neurotic repetitions from the past. The patient's transference was conceived of as an objective fact.

Notice how this formulation assumes that if the patient were in analysis with any one of ten well-trained, competent analysts, the patient's transference would be the same. It took many decades before analysts began to challenge this formulation. In retrospect it seems obvious that the gender, physical appearance, age, manner of speaking, office décor, missed session policy, skin color, accent, and degree of interactivity of the analyst would have some effect on the patient's transference. In addition to all these factors, the therapist's countertransference would likely have the greatest effect on the patient's transference, as later examples in this chapter will illustrate.

The field of psychotherapy has come a long way. In one of the seismic shifts in psychological theory, today's zeitgeist of intersubjectivity posits that what transpires during the therapy hour is co-constructed by the therapist and patient. Ten different therapists treating the same patient would inevitably produce ten somewhat different outcomes—maybe a little different or a lot different depending on the particular therapist. The classical idea maintained that countertransference could and should be kept out of the therapy, but if it wasn't, the therapist's feelings had a deleterious effect on the therapy. The therapist was to get supervision or possibly even therapy. Notice how this formulation doesn't allow for the possibility that the therapist's feelings or personal experiences could have a positive effect on the therapy. The modern notion of countertransference understands that it will inevitably find its way into the therapy but that this is not bad. What can be

DOI: 10.4324/9781003174608-4

harmful is when the therapist is either not aware of the intrusion of countertransference or not receptive to working with it when it is pointed out. Put positively, countertransference can be employed for therapeutic purposes.

Let's consider one example. Assume that the patient and therapist have worked hard and productively over a 5-year period and the patient has resolved a career-limiting problem with authority and harsh self-criticism. The patient begins noting her frequent thoughts about terminating her therapy in its fifth year. Patient and therapist agree to devote the next 3 months to exploring this wish to ensure that what is decided is in the best interest of the patient. Let's also assume that the patient is ready to terminate.

It turns out that the patient's therapist, also a woman, happens to have unresolved issues with being left. She is unaware of this blind spot. Instead of being able to acknowledge and hopefully even celebrate the patient's impressive work in therapy, the therapist acts as if she is being abandoned. Her reactions to the patient's progress are stilted. Her mild but persistent skepticism about her patient's wish to terminate create sporadic moments of self-doubt in her patient. Even so, her patient's confidence about her own judgment prevails and she decides to terminate. The sense of trust and safety that she has felt with her therapist feels slightly tarnished as she terminates her therapy. She is uncertain if she would return to this therapist should the need arise.

Now consider another therapist who treats this same patient. As in the first therapy, the patient and therapist work effectively for 5 years and the patient resolves her issues with authority and harsh self-criticism. After 5 years of therapy, the patient feels ready to terminate and they agree to give the termination process 3 months. This therapist happens to have three daughters, two of whom have already left home and are in college. Letting go emotionally has been difficult but now with the third daughter ready to leave for college, the therapist—and his wife—feel ready. They truly celebrate their youngest daughter's achievements and feel ready to embrace whatever the empty nest has in store for them. This male therapist's response to his patient's well-earned desire to terminate is colored by his experience with his youngest daughter. He feels excitement for her and is able to celebrate her accomplishments in therapy. Riding home in his car after their final session, he again realizes that that his patient reminds him in some ways of his youngest daughter. As the patient leaves the therapy, she knows that should she have any difficulty in the future she would return to this therapist.

The example I just provided is a rather glaring example of the statement "There are no completely objective data in interpersonal relations. The way I am with you partly determines the way you are with me." More *subtle* examples of this phenomenon are common in everyday practice. Despite efforts that therapists make to ensure that they are not impeding the very therapy they are trying to advance, they inevitably and occasionally fall short of this goal. Here is a personal example.

A patient said to me: "Dr. Gans, I notice that when I pay my bill late you usually ask me if I have any thoughts about the late payment. However, when I pay my bill immediately you never ask if I have any thoughts about my promptness."

"What thoughts or feelings do you have about my inconsistency?" I asked. He answered, " Since you could probably learn as much about me by inquiring about my paying immediately as you can by asking me about my paying late, I get the feeling that your only asking about my paying late is not about an effort on your part to know more about me but more about wanting to make sure you get paid." "How do your observations affect your feelings about me?" I asked. "I trust you," he said, "but from something you once mentioned about your father, I think you have some issues about money."

Another subtle example of the statement came up while I was supervising a therapist. She reported that she was five minutes late to an appointment with her patient and immediately said, "I can make up the five minutes at the end of the session." Her patient—who at the time had negative feelings toward her therapist—replied: "Why didn't you say that you would make up the five minutes if I [the patient] can or wanted to? What if I don't want to make up the five minutes, something you might not find out about in assuming that I would." The therapist's well-intentioned but somewhat insensitive comment added to her patient's negative transference.

The radical shift in psychological theory from a one-person psychology where one person's subjectivity is the object of study to a two-person psychology where two subjectivities interact has assigned an additional task to therapists: the constant need to keep in mind that their way of relating to the patient partly determines how the patient will relate to them.[1]

Note

1 Stark, M. (2000). *Modes of therapeutic action.* Lanham, MD: Roman & Littlefield.

Chapter 2

Many natural reactions are not helpful and many helpful reactions do not come naturally.

Marilyn was a 36-year-old, married mother of two teenage daughters. She was a childhood diabetic who resented all the restrictions her disease had imposed on her. She had many unresolved issues with her alternately remote and intrusive mother. She married young and her alcoholic husband was physically and emotionally abusive. She enjoyed her work as an office manager for a physician, partly because the job got her out of the home and away from her husband who was out of work and at home on temporary disability. Weekends were hell. Between one daughter's defiance and acting-out and her husband's drinking and disparaging comments, she at times felt hopeless and suicidal. She had a brief erotic, psychotic episode after work when she began taking her clothes off in front of the physician she was working for, believing her boss was in love with her.

I saw Marilyn for weekly 50-minute sessions on Friday afternoons. As the session was ending at 5:20 (my last appointment of the week), Marilyn would invariably wish me a "very nice weekend." It became painfully clear—at least to me—that I was going to have a very much nicer weekend than Marilyn was going to have. I found myself falling into the *natural* and customary pattern of wishing her one as well. This natural reaction was not useful because it didn't help her get at the bitterness and resentment that resided beneath her good manners. Her parting comment was more appropriate for friendship than an in-depth psychotherapy designed to promote introspection and self-awareness. As I gradually became aware that her parting comment—now a ritual—contained unexpressed feelings toward me, I was able to bring to her attention the session-ending pattern that had emerged. She was eventually able to speak of her envy of my (imagined) situation, a disclosure that freed her up to speak of several concerns that she had not previously brought into therapy.

The preceding example illustrates how easily therapists can get pulled into socially conditioned responses. We are social animals and therefore react in socially conditioned ways. As therapists we need to maintain a fine balance between being socially appropriate and being curious. The challenge is to bring the patient's attention to the evolving social ritual in such a way that we enlist their curiosity while not shaming them or appearing rude.

DOI: 10.4324/9781003174608-5

It is natural to want to cover up one's mistakes, but for a therapist to do so in therapy is a clinical mistake, as the following example illustrates. The example also illustrates how the therapist, acting unnaturally, can sometimes be useful to the patient.

A single man in his early 50s, John entered therapy recounting a series of failed heterosexual relationships and despaired about ever having a permanent, stable relationship. Twenty minutes into the first session held at my home office, he became aware that his beloved dog that he had left in his truck was barking. He seemed unnerved by the barking and was about to go out and check on his dog when I casually mentioned that the barking was coming from two German Shepherds owned by one of my across-the-street neighbors. Ignoring my comment, John temporarily left the session to check. John had "read" his dog's emotional state correctly, sensing that his dog was in distress. John had suspected that by contagion his dog had taken on some of the great anxiety with which John approached this initial session. John returned to the session, distraught on two accounts: (1) his highly agitated dog, his closest companion, had responded to the abandonment by tearing up the inside of John's truck, and (2) equally upsetting, John reacted negatively to what he took to be my presumptuousness. While it was my intention to reassure John that the barking dogs were nothing to worry about, John took the remark to indicate that I had no clue about his closeness to his dog. From John's point of view, if the therapist had not already gleaned that simple and important fact, how could the therapist understand anything else that was important about him? It was immediately clear that if this therapy was to continue, I would need to own my empathic failure and certainly not try to do what was *natural*, namely, to explain how unlikely it was that anyone would, in the short period of time and with the amount of data provided, have had any way of knowing how close John and his dog were.

Several additional sessions seemed to reassure John that we could work productively together. Several years into the therapy I made another mistake, this one more benign. John, who had previously been in a number of alternative therapies including transcendental meditation, came into a session and said that he wanted to use the remaining 40 minutes to meditate. While this was a very unusual request in my clinical experience, I felt, for a variety of reasons—hopefully for John's benefit—that I should go along with his request. His session was the last one of my day near the end of what had been an exhausting week. He closed his eyes and, without my realizing it, mine closed as well. More worn-out than I appreciated, John's eyes-closed, meditative state lulled me into sleep. When I woke up it was two minutes after the 50-minute session should have ended; John *appeared* to be in a deep meditative state. The next week there was no mention of what had transpired during the previous week's session.

I began our session a few weeks later saying that I needed to talk with him about an administrative matter. John appeared apprehensive. Having had time to metabolize a variety of feelings that the situation had stirred up in me, I explained that while it was his prerogative to use therapy time in any constructive fashion he desired, it was my job to be present and awake during the session. I calculated the monetary value of how long I had been asleep and said I owed him that amount. It turned out that John had noted that I had been asleep but had never mentioned it. For John, who had profound feelings of distrust of his parents, especially his father, my handling of this situation, *although it certainly did not come naturally*, proved to be therapeutic and enhanced John's trust in the process and in me.

Readers familiar with psychotherapy and its language—be they therapists or patients—will recognize that the statement "Many helpful reactions do not come naturally" refers to how therapists' manage—or "metabolize"—the effects that patients exert on them, including difficult to manage situations that arise between them.

Here is an account of many urges, thoughts, and feelings I had to metabolize before I could decide how to deal therapeutically with this situation. First, I had to deal with my feelings about whether John actually had noticed that I had been asleep. At first glance it seemed to me that he hadn't, even though I thought he might have. Should I proceed as if I had been awake and attentive during the last 40 minutes of the session or should I be honest about the fact that I was asleep myself? My first reaction in dealing with these two possibilities had to do with my own father and his stance toward money. A middleman in the fruit business with a fourth-grade education, his greatest pleasure seemed to be getting the better of the other guy in a business transaction. Having internalized some of my father's ways of doing business, some of which crossed a line, I had to confront my corrupt impulses.

As I was thinking that I shouldn't get paid for time that I hadn't worked, it occurred to me that if my father had been in that situation, there was no way he would have refunded part of what John had paid for the session. Part of me didn't want to either. But I knew that if I indulged my dishonest impulses, I wouldn't feel good about myself. Second, given that John had parents he didn't trust, I appreciated how very important it was for him to have a therapist who was honest and trustworthy. Third, I knew that my values differed from my father's—partly made possible by a life more comfortable than his—and I wanted to do the right thing. Without judging my father, I knew what was the right thing to do.

Then the question arose, how do I handle the situation in a way that would have the most therapeutic value for John? I found myself associating to one of his recurrent dreams. A large bird with talons sat on his left shoulder. Any time John moved, the bird's talons ripped his flesh. The dream captured how immobilized with fear John felt when his father called him into the living room "to have a talk." During such meetings his father would administer harsh punishments for minor infractions. The dread that John felt with his father resurfaced in routine meetings with people in positions of authority.

The following idea came to me: if after a few sessions went by and John did not bring up the session in question, I would tell him that I wanted to speak to him about an administrative matter. I thought that what I had to tell him would contrast sharply with what he anticipated I had to say. He would expect bad news and I would deliver good news. I thought his heightened affect around such a discussion would help him see how hard it was for him to give other people the benefit of the doubt or trust other people—an aspect of himself that he felt badly about. As I told him about the refund and the reasons why, the expression on his face contained many feelings that we had weeks to process.

Chapter 3

With some patients there is no *risk* of ever establishing the truth.

When I arrived at Massachusetts Mental Health Center in July 1968 to begin my psychiatric residency, I was smarter than I would ever be again. I was fresh out of my internship in internal medicine, filled with all manner of medical information: disease states, medications, treatment regimens, differential diagnoses, and physical signs and symptoms and their significance. What a shock to realize that hardly any of this information was going to be useful in helping psychotic patients who populated the hospital wards where I trained. Even though internship had taught me ways to appraise through inspection alone how physically ill a patient is—pallor, rapid respirations, jaundice, massively swollen legs—I now realized, as a psychiatric resident, that I did not know how to estimate the degree of psychological illness. Is the person healthy, sick, very sick, or very, very sick psychologically? Finding out the emotional truth of a person's experience was to prove more complex than having a vast fund of medical information.

Psychiatric training provided ways of thinking about emotional illness. One approach involved thinking about basic tasks of living: survival, getting others to do things for us, and maintaining relationships we already have. Preoccupation with one or another of these tasks provides clues to how sick someone is psychologically. People struggling with survival are on the sickest end of the spectrum while people maintaining relationships that they already have are on the healthier end of the spectrum.

Certain psychological mechanisms of defense, some of them unconscious, are associated with these various tasks. People struggling with survival employ primarily projection, distortion, denial, and projective identification. People attempting to get others to do things for them utilize hypochondriasis ("if you don't love me at least you can pay attention to my elbow, it's killing me"), characterological depression, anxiety, and astute ineptness. People attempting to maintain relationships that they already have employ higher level functions such as humor, planning, altruism, generosity, kindness, etc. Thus, by observing the ego functions primarily utilized, one can extrapolate back to the basic tasks of living with which they are preoccupied and, by this line of reasoning, estimate the degree of their emotional health or sickness.[1]

Yet even with the most sophisticated approaches to assessing and working with psychological dysfunction, there are some patients with whom there seems to be

DOI: 10.4324/9781003174608-6

no risk of establishing factual, not to mention emotional, truth, as the following example illustrates.

A nurse and daughter of a physician, Catherine was a 44-year-old mother of one teenage son. She was referred for psychiatric treatment by her internist who believed that her illnesses—multiple and very serious infections—were self-inflicted. It was unclear whether she had an immunologic deficiency that predisposed her to multiple infections or if she had a serious case of factitious illness, or both. As the patient put it, "If I'm not doing this to myself, I must have a terrible immunologic deficiency; if I am doing this to myself and I'm not aware that I am, that realization shakes the whole foundation of my sense of myself."

Catherine's infections involved her skin, breasts, neck, bones, kidneys, uterus, and vagina. Early in the treatment, an infectious disease consultant informed her that she had an underlying immunological—IgG—deficiency which predisposed her to recurrent infections. During the 10 years I treated Catherine with weekly psychotherapy, she had 20 surgeries, was treated by 12 different physicians, and was prescribed 25 medications. She evoked polar reactions from her surgeons; some opted for heroic measures while others wanted no part of ever treating her again. In psychotherapy, she evidenced little capacity for introspection. I received several calls from physicians who pressed me on whether I thought she was causing these illnesses to herself.

I essentially took the position that I was her therapist, not a detective, and that I was trying to help her cope with her overwhelming physical and emotional pain. It was clear that her managed care company would not be unhappy if she died, as she was a huge financial drain. I tried to keep in my mind the infectious disease consultant's report indicating that she did have a biological disorder. On the other hand, psychological data such as misusing psychotropic medication, blaming doctors and playing one off against the other, evoking distrust in her medical and surgical caregivers, and using guilt-induction as a weapon—"you will feel sorry at my funeral"—suggested that emotional factors played a significant role in her suffering. And if her condition was predominantly psychologically generated, her bland willingness to undergo a mastectomy—to sacrifice a body part as a substitute solution for dealing with a psychological conflict—was truly impressive in its self-destructiveness. Later in our treatment another infectious disease consultant suggested that the bacteria *Escherichia coli* was the cause of all of Catherine's infections. This consultant hypothesized that Catherine was injecting fecally contaminated water into various parts of her body. It was no wonder that I was confused about the etiology of her recurrent infections.

So, where did I locate Catherine on the continuum of mental health and mental illness? One the one hand, she had been married for 22 years, had a child, and worked as a nurse. She did have an immunologic deficiency that predisposed her to infections that interfered with her parenting and her work as a nurse. She came to therapy faithfully for 10 years and was not psychotic. On the other hand, during her adult life she had had 20 surgeries for self-induced infections in a variety of organs. She elicited polar opposite emotional reactions in the many physicians that cared for her, although almost all finally resigned from her case in frustration or disgust. It seemed that her solution to dealing with unacceptable emotional longings or conflict was to sacrifice a body part to obtain concern from her family and attention from the medical community. While estimations of psychopathology are never precise, I located Catherine as being somewhere between being very sick and very, very sick emotionally.

One day I received a call from her pharmacist. He asked me if I had a habit of doodling when I wrote prescriptions. I asked him what he meant. He said that on a prescription for 1 milligram of lorazepam that I had written for Catherine, the 1 was written over and now appeared as a 2. He thought she had tampered with the prescription and faxed it to me.

Finally, I thought to myself, I have proof that Catherine is not to be trusted with prescriptions I write for her, or as an accurate and reliable historian. In our next appointment after the call I received from the pharmacist, I said to her: "Up to this point in the therapy I have taken the position that I don't know if you are causing these infections or not—despite the many physicians who believe that you are. I have felt that it is my job to deal with your suffering and to provide support. But yesterday I got a call from your pharmacist. I have elected to take what I learned from him as a form of supervision. I wonder if his call is your indirect way of indicating that I should focus more on your unreliability." She asked what I meant. I showed her the copy of the prescription and asked her if she had made that alteration. She gave me a priceless answer, "If I did that I must be a very sick person." I asked, "Did you?" to which she answered, "I don't think so." I was so taken aback by her answer that I didn't have the presence of mind to say, "Are you worried that if you are that sick I'll decide not be your doctor anymore?" This interaction taught me that with some people there is no *risk* of ever establishing the truth.

Note

1 Rako, S., & Mazer, H. (1980). *Semrad: The heart of a therapist*. New York: Jason Aronson, pp. 155–156.

Chapter 4

In most cases, all things being considered, people are doing the best they can. If you don't think so, you probably don't have enough information or you do not fully understand the information you do have.

In his short story, "A Face of Stone," William Carlos Williams beautifully depicts his judgments about a family he is treating which he instantly dislikes.[1] They are pushy, and feel self-entitled to boot. Imagining them to be Italian immigrants, he is put off by the wife's expressionless face. She is dirty, smelly, unrestrained, obstinate, and unintelligent. His first thoughts were, "People like that belong in clinics" and "We should keep them out of the country." The wife frantically holds on to her child whom she believes is sick, despite the lack of any objective evidence. Her husband lovingly explains to Dr Williams that his wife is new to this country and is afraid that he, the doctor, will hurt her baby. They want reassurances from the doctor that he will be available night or day, should the need arise. The doctor bristles at their sense of self-importance. Dr Williams observes the woman with disdain and disgust, noting her broken English, her decayed teeth, ruptured varicose veins, bowed lower legs "that could not have come from anything but severe rickets in her late childhood," her torn dress, and fractured English. Dr Williams asks the husband the age of his wife and is shocked to learn that she is only 24. When Dr Williams learns that this woman lost her entire family in the Holocaust, had little food to eat during the war—the reason for her dental caries and her bowed legs—and is now totally consumed with the health of her baby, he is filled with shame over his tone of voice, dismissive attitude, and his arrogant presumptuousness.

Dr Williams' reactions are an extreme version of what not infrequently occurs in therapy when therapists become impatient with their patients' lack of progress.

Sometimes it's only after therapists have organized their patient's history in a time framework that they become better able to understand why their patient is in fact doing the best he/she can. Compare these two versions of Mr N's history, the first presented ahistorically, the second in a time framework.

Mr N, a 59-year-old married father of seven, is himself the oldest of three boys whose parents divorced. His youngest brother died as an infant. The patient's father moved him and his middle brother from Massachusetts to New York shortly thereafter. He kept in touch with his mother who remained in Massachusetts. He

DOI: 10.4324/9781003174608-7

finished high school and spent 4 years in the Navy. After working as a machinist, he married a recently widowed woman who had three children, and they settled in Massachusetts. Mr N and his wife then had four children of their own. The patient's mother is living and his father, who had drinking problems, died after the patient had relocated him to a Massachusetts nursing home. During the first 16 years of his marriage, he had bought 20 automobiles, none of which ever satisfied him. He came to therapy complaining of depression.

Not keeping the events of a patient's life and symptom formation in a time framework can obscure the overwhelming life challenges a patient is facing. Without a time framework, a patient's history does not come to life. Conversely, viewing the patient's history chronologically puts flesh and blood to what otherwise might remain a string of seemingly unrelated events. Suddenly a palpable human being's falling ill becomes quite understandable—and compelling. Here is a retelling of Mr N's history put in a time framework.

Year	Age	Event
1906		Father born
1907		Mother born
1924		Mr N born (parents 18 and 17)
1928	4	Middle brother born
1931	7	Youngest brother born
1932	8	Youngest brother dies at 11 months; parents' marriage breaking up
1933	9	Parents divorce; mother given custody
1934	10	Father takes patient and brother and settles in New York state; patient keeps in touch with mother in Massachusetts
1942	18	Patient graduates high school
1942–1946	18–22	Serves in the Navy for 4 years
1946–1963	22–39	Works as a machinist; several unhappy love affairs; leads carefree life
1963	39	Marries a widow with children ages 9, 8, 7
1964–1969	40–45	Settles in Massachusetts and has 4 children
1976	52	Brings 70-year-old father with strokes and an alcohol problem from New York to Massachusetts, places him a nursing home; father dies 3 months later
1963–1979	39–55	Bought 20 automobiles during this time period, none of which satisfy

Organizing the patient's story in a time framework highlights the relationships among life events that might otherwise have been glossed over or missed. Grasping the likely significance of certain life events, the therapist can ask questions that invite the patient to elaborate. For example, during the Depression, when Mr N was between the ages of eight and ten, he was dealing with the recent death of his youngest brother, his parents' divorce, and separation from his mother. Asking him what he remembered during those times would likely provide formative memories regarding emotional survival and coping skills. What might the therapist inquire about after noticing that from ages 39–45, Mr N went from being carefree and single for 17 years to being married with seven children? What was coping with all that new responsibility like for him? Was the decision to have four children, in addition to three from his wife's previous marriage, a mutual decision? How did he manage to continue caring for his alcoholic father when he had so much family responsibility? With all the children to support, was there any resentment on his wife's part about his purchase of 20 automobiles over a 16-year period? Keeping in mind Mr N's early losses and separation from his mother, the therapist could validate his many strengths: staying in touch with his mother, graduating high school, functioning in the military, and moving his elderly father to be closer to his family.

Keeping Mr N's story in a time framework helps in the construction of a psychodynamic formulation.[2] Born to very young parents, ages 18 and 17, the patient's early life during the Depression was traumatic—a sibling's death, parental divorce, separation from his mother, all occurring between the ages of 8 and 10. Disappointed, conflicted, and probably guilty over his parent's divorce and sibling's death, he nevertheless possessed sufficient strength to keep in touch with his mother, graduate from high school, and function well in the military. Hurt and frightened by family life, he had "fun" as a single person for 17 years while he avoided dealing with his inner conflicts. *Over the next 6 years, from ages 39 to 45, Mr N went from being carefree and single to being married with seven children!* He unconsciously tried to solve his inner fears about his family experience by creating the home he yearned for but had never had. Instead of securing the fantasized "perfect family," this faulty solution saddled him with massive responsibilities that overwhelmed and drained him. He began to identify with his sickly father who died shortly thereafter. He began to resent having to give to his children all that he never received. Even the compulsive buying of 20 cars over 16 years could not provide him pleasure. He ended up feeling like a sibling to his children and the least favored by his wife. In this context he became depressed and sought out therapy.

Notes

1 William, W. C. (1984). *The Doctor Stories*. New York City: The New Directions Publishing Corporation.
2 Perry, S., Cooper, A. M., & Michels, R. (1987). The psychodynamic formulation: Its purpose, structure, and clinical application. *Am J of Psychiatry*, 144: 543–550.

Chapter 5

It is at the boundaries that meaningful psychotherapeutic work takes place.

Medical professionals require protection to do their work safely. Dentists wear gloves. Surgeons wear masks and gowns. Radiologists wear lead aprons. The protection that these professionals employ provides safety for their patients as well. Psychotherapists also require some sort of protection both to contain and detoxify the powerful emotional forces that invariably arise in the course of psychotherapy. Boundaries provide needed protection for both patient and therapist.[1]

The treatment frame is one type of boundary. It comprises the who, what, where, when, and why of the work. The therapist is the designated helper and the patient is the person seeking help. They agree to meet in a certain place, the therapist's office, for a certain period of time, usually 45 or 50 minutes/week, with a given frequency, often weekly, and on a given day of the week. The patient agrees to pay a fee determined by the therapist if the patient is paying privately; the therapist agrees to accept the reimbursement fee set by the insurance company if the patient is using insurance that the provider has agreed to accept. It is understood that what takes place in the sessions is confidential, except in very infrequent and special situations. Except for situations that involve imminent danger or when the patient gives the therapist permission to talk with other people, the therapist agrees to treat the patient based on only what the patient tells the therapist. The purpose of the treatment is to help the patient get a better understanding of the forces in the past and present that have contributed to the problems for which help is sought. Both parties agree to hold themselves responsible and abide by these agreements.

When therapist and patient agree upon these ground rules, they form a durable container in which the work of psychotherapy can take place safely. The therapist's dependability, consistency and reliability, along with compassionate, non-judgmental listening, solidify the initial sense of safety that the framework of therapy provides. As earned trust is established, patients' stories spill out: the effects of a bitter parental divorce; an abortion performed by a physician husband that was not talked about for 15 years; what it was like to grow up in a home run like a military camp; the anguish involved in dealing with a drug addicted child; the lasting effects of sexual abuse; the inaccessibility of a narcissistic parent.

The therapist listens and relates as a participant observer. In the initial phase of therapy, the therapist attends in a particular way. Aware that there are many

DOI: 10.4324/9781003174608-8

ways of thinking about the story the patient relates, the therapist takes an accepting stance toward the patient's narrative. At the same time, the therapist makes a number of observations, some of which take boundary matters into consideration.

The therapist pays special attention to the first topic with which the patient begins the session. The therapist appreciates that the patient had to select that topic from an almost infinite number of possibilities. Because of this selection process, the topic selected often has special significance inasmuch as it has "won out" over all the other topics that might have been selected. Often such material is not random. It has prevailed because it is striving for recognition. Here is an example. Phyllis began her first session upon returning from her vacation in Italy by talking in an extended fashion about her fellow travelers and how much more money they had to spend than she did. I knew that she had been on a tight budget for the trip. I began to wonder why I wasn't hearing about the Swiss Alps, Lake Como, Italian food, or her cousins whom she and her husband were visiting in Rome. I noted that there was less eye contact than usual. It occurred to me that we were meeting on the seventh day of the month and that she had probably just gotten her monthly bill from me. I bill at the end of the month and expect payment within a month. Sure enough, she was angry that I had not been able to fill her session while she was away, a session for which she knew she could be charged. Although we had gone over it several times before, she had conveniently forgotten her knowledge of and agreement with my policy for missed sessions. Discussing that topic led to the resurfacing of feelings of deprivation in childhood that had more to do with emotional than financial deprivation. In this example, my missed session policy constituted a boundary that Phyllis had agreed to, forgotten about, and now objected to. We agreed to put the financial question on the back burner and attend first to the emotional issues that had been stirred up.

Therapists similarly pay attention to what transpires around another boundary, namely, the ending of a session.[2] If for no other reason, emotional disclosures made at the end of a session are important because there is no time to explore their possible significance. The ending of a session can be thought of as a recurrent mini-separation that can revive memories of separations in both patient and therapist. Separations are one of the more powerful emotional phenomena that human beings deal with. Some examples include: early separations from one's mother or first primary caretaker; starting school; forming ideas different from ones strongly held by one's parents; leaving home; getting married, etc. Separations that have been experienced as or actually are abandonments leave life-long scars. People wonder if during such separations they will be kept in mind by the important people in their lives, as the following example illustrates.

I saw Evelyn in weekly group psychotherapy and every other week in individual therapy. Six months into her therapy, Evelyn made a serious suicide attempt. By the end of the first year of treatment a strong connection with Evelyn had been made in both treatments. After 15 months of treatment and two weeks before my three-week vacation—which as usual I had announced a month in advance—Evelyn announced at the end of a group session that she was again feeling suicidal. Group members appeared very concerned and immediately looked to me for some direction. I looked at the group and said, "It will be difficult for us not to keep Evelyn in mind until our next meeting and also to end this meeting on time."

Before the final group meeting before vacation, Evelyn and I met in our scheduled individual appointment. She alluded to my comment at the end of the previous group session and said that she had been comforted by it. My comment clarified an intention that she was barely aware of in making the suicidal declaration. In the best way available to her at the time, she wanted reassurance that her connection with the group was not in peril. She had realized that she needed their ongoing concern and attention that she valued during the time the group would not be meeting. My comment addressed her fear and worry that she was wearing the group down with her relentless feelings of hopelessness and that we were getting tired of her—which I didn't think was the case. She correctly understood that my intent in making the comment was to let her know that we would be keeping her in mind when the group wasn't meeting.

Remembering that it is at the boundaries that important therapeutic work often takes places helped me to think of other meanings or intentions that might have resided in the timing of her suicidal declaration. The boundaries involved in this example include the impending end of the session, my upcoming vacation, and the line between unconscious motivation and conscious recognition. By ending on time the session in which she made her suicidal comment and by understanding her unconscious motivation, I provided the safety needed until I met with Evelyn in an individual session.

Group therapy highlights another important boundary, namely, what takes place inside the session as compared to what takes place outside of the session. The framework of therapy is designed to create a distinctive space—one that differs from ordinary social interaction—where the participants dedicate themselves to personal and interpersonal learning and to open and honest communication. People expect themselves and the others to be authentic and spontaneous rather than polite or nice. Unreasonable feelings are welcomed in the service of personal growth. Efforts are made to re-own projected feelings that might result in scapegoating. The possible meanings of where people sit and how people speak are examined. Group members slowly realize that they can't say something about another group member without revealing something about themselves. An example from my group therapy practice highlights the significance of this boundary as an indicator of the amount of therapeutic work a particular patient has completed.

Tom was very friendly, talkative, and good-natured in the waiting room. From what group members reported, his behavior and his way of relating during the group sessions did not differ much from his behavior in the waiting room. After seven months in the group and abiding by a norm in the group contract that specified "I agree to allow the group to participate in my decision to terminate," Tom good-naturedly, and to the group's surprise, invited feedback about his intention to leave group. Evelyn pointed out that there was no difference in Tom's way of relating inside and outside of the group. Tom asked innocently why that observation was significant. In a show of unanimity infrequent in group therapy where there are usually several different reactions to a given group occurrence, Fred, acting as a spokesman for the group said, "If you don't understand the difference between what goes on in the waiting room and in the therapy office, there is no way that you are ready to leave. Actually, you're just beginning the process." Sasha said, "In the waiting room we talk about the weather, good movies we've seen, just idle chit-chat. In the office we reveal things that are difficult and how the problems we're having with each other might be related to the difficulties that brought each one of us into therapy." Here the group was trying to educate Tom about the group as a sacred space where people dedicate themselves to the hard work of learning about themselves and the "other," not to mention issues of power, control, mutuality, sibling, and authority issues, etc. Tom listened intently to the feedback but, sadly, seemed satisfied with his group experience and decided to leave the group.

Another set of less visible boundaries plays an important role in managing the strong emotional currents that arise as psychotherapeutic work deepens. These boundaries are interpersonal and intrapsychic. For the therapist to participate in the patient's feelings, there needs to be permeability in the boundary that separates the therapist and the patient. If the boundary is too permeable, a sense of over-identification or merger might occur that could frighten both parties and confuse whose material is whose. If the boundary is impermeable, the therapist is unable to experience the patient emotionally, to get a feel for the patient's inner world. Moreover, if the boundary between the therapist's conscious and unconscious mind is too impermeable, the therapist will be limited in his ability to access associations and fantasies to the patient's productions. If that boundary is too permeable, the therapist, overwhelmed by a rush of internal associations, may lose his/her therapeutic balance and focus. Countertransference difficulties result. Here is an example.

Paul, a 45-year-old man married for 18 years, enters twice weekly therapy with a male therapist, Norman, his own age. They meet in Norman's home office. Paul's history is notable for the fact that his parents divorced when he was 16, tarnishing what he thought was a happy childhood. The patient has two teen-age daughters, one of whom has been acting out sexually. The daughters, one year apart, will have left for college in two years. Paul has been having sleepless nights and arguments with his wife about how best to manage their daughter's behavior. Paul's wife, Diane, has put her career as an architect on hold to raise the children, is somewhat depressed and, recently, unresponsive sexually. Paul, on the other hand, is a very successful entrepreneur whose business now almost runs itself. Paul's shiny, new red Porsche sits parked outside Norman's modest home.

After six months in therapy, Paul reveals that he has been having an affair with a 30-year-old single woman who is starting her own business. Paul describes the woman, Betsy, as brilliant, incredibly attractive, a great cook, and terrific in bed. Paul starts missing sessions—which he gladly pays for—because of outings with Betsy, many of them in her bedroom.

Norman notices several reactions he has begun to have toward Paul. He is sufficiently titillated by Paul's graphic descriptions of sex with Betsy that he fails to ask questions such as, "Why do you think you are sharing all these details with me?" Or, "How did you imagine I would respond to this information?" Or, "How would you like me to respond to this disclosure—and why?" Sexually activated by Paul's stories, Norman begins to express concerns about Paul's infidelity and starts to caution Paul about the slippery slope he may be on instead of exploring with Paul how he might be feeling in general—and, later, about his feelings about his wife and daughters. [Notice how Paul could be feeling at this point in therapy, "Why am I paying for advice that I could easily be getting from well-meaning friends?"] Norman also fails to explore how Paul remembers feeling around the time of his parents' divorce. Over-stimulated sexually by Paul's accounts of his sexual escapades, Norman becomes threatened and preoccupied with his own sexual impulses, exacerbated by the lack of sex he is having at home. He unconsciously projects his activated sexual fantasies on to Paul and, believing his projections, experiences Paul to be more infatuated with Betsy than Paul experiences himself to be.

The combination of Norman's threatened sexuality and his preoccupation with Paul's acting-out weakens Norman's connection to his patient. There are at least two therapeutic causalities that result from the rupture of the therapeutic bond. The connections of Paul's affair to his daughter's sexual acting out, to his wife's sexual withdrawal, and to his parents' divorce are not explored. Second, the therapy itself is threatened as Paul begins to feel that he is getting more out his relationship with Betsy than he is from his therapy. Unfortunately, Norman comes to these realizations too late and Paul suddenly and unilaterally leaves the therapy.

Notes

1 Gabbard, G. O., & Lester, E. P. (1995). *Boundaries and Boundary Violations in Psychoanalysis*. New York: Basic Books.
2 Gans, J. S. (2016). "Our time is up": A relational perspective on the ending of a single psychotherapy session. *Am J Psychother*, 70: 413–427.

Chapter 6

In chronic marital discord, each partner is contributing approximately 50% of the problem no matter how asymmetrically they present or seem during the course of the therapy.

In couple therapy, the therapist must be empathically attuned to each member of the couple. This compassionate neutrality is the glue that helps both spouses feel like valued, worthwhile people, and keeps each working on their contributions to the chronic marital difficulties. However, the confusing nature of couple therapy combined with therapists' inexperience often results in taking sides. If the therapist *permanently* takes the side of one partner the therapy will fail. The therapist must be aware of this dynamic and strive to return to compassionate neutrality as the therapy unfolds.

The therapist's compassionate neutrality has many components. Here is a partial list:

- helping each partner feel understood, respected, and empathized with;
- feeling touched by each partner's story and, failing that, trying to understand why;
- indicating an interest in collaborating with rather than in doing something to, for, or on the couple;
- remembering that couples originally got together because they found qualities in each other that they valued, and inquiring about these qualities;
- keeping in mind that partners complain about each other because they are not receiving the emotional responsiveness they need;
- appreciating that some of the deprivation that partners experience at the hands of each other actually existed in each of them before they met and were attracted to each other;
- entertaining the possibility that in marrying, the partners unconsciously hoped that this institution would be the solution to feelings of childhood neglect or abuse;
- realizing that many unconscious forces at play cannot yet be comprehended.

These components of the therapist's compassionate neutrality serve to oppose the forces that threaten to tear the marriage apart. That said, the *major* goal of compassionate neutrality is not the saving of the marriage. The major goal is that each member of the couple be able to live the fullest life possible.

DOI: 10.4324/9781003174608-9

Once the therapist's compassionate neutrality gets short-circuited and is replaced by permanent side taking, the lesser valued partner often feels devalued, scapegoated, and less interested in attending the sessions. The therapy may end and the marriage may be put further in jeopardy. Conversely, the therapist's ability and determination to maintain compassionate neutrality while appreciating that each member of the couple contributes an equal amount to its difficulties allows the therapy to take hold and proceed. This even-handed approach of the therapist is difficult to accomplish. Many factors make it hard for the therapist to proceed on the notion that members of the marriage are equally responsible for their marital difficulties.

The first reason that the therapist can lose sight of the equal contributions of each partner to the couple's chronic marital difficulties is that the couple usually presents asymmetrically. One person, often the wife, who speaks the feeling-filled language of psychotherapy, describes her husband as being very difficult (unfeeling, passive, or abusive). She appears to be a nice person who has been mistreated or neglected. Obviously one person is at fault here. It doesn't appear to be a 50–50 proposition. Seasoned couple therapists appreciate that spouses who present as devils and angels often turn out to be unwitting co-conspirators. For example, a husband's passivity, meekness, and low self-esteem emerge as facilitators of his wife's chronic sense of entitlement and resulting affairs. Simply blaming her absolves her husband of the responsibility to grow and change. First impressions can be powerful and difficult to fully overcome.

A second reason why it doesn't seem that each partner is contributing equally to the marital problems has to do with the sex of the therapist. The therapist's gender stereotypes may impede the therapist's maintenance of compassionate neutrality. Female therapists often find the husband to be insensitive, overly passive, and inexperienced or disinterested in dealing with feelings. Male couple therapists—a seemingly rare breed these days—often have an unusual facility "for a man" for dealing with feelings and may want to help the husband in that area. Thus, the female therapist may be more on the side of the wife and the male therapist more on the side of the husband. An exception to this pattern arises when a member of the couple is especially attractive or seductive in which case the therapist is pulled to bond with the member of the couple of the opposite sex. Once again, it doesn't feel like a 50–50 deal to the therapist.

A third reason is that the therapist may initially believe one spouse is more responsible for the couple's problems. The therapist may buy into a common contention in couple therapy, namely, that the other spouse "was not like this before we married." Each member of the couple can be very persuasive in making this contention and, in the process, make it difficult for the therapist to keep an open mind. It goes something like this: "She was very understanding when I met her and now she is so controlling." Or, "He was sensitive and caring and now he is self-absorbed and always working." She might add that her husband, like so many men, has the "delusion" that he is just a nice guy. It seems like each member of the couple was the victim of false advertising. This contention sometimes overlooks the fact that not much has really changed in each spouse before and after they married, if only each one had noticed certain telltale signs in the other. Some examples that the therapist can elicit or that the couple relates over time include: the person was always late, hadn't separated emotionally from his/her family of origin, apologized immediately in arguments thereby short-circuiting real conversations, couldn't/wouldn't own his/her part in an argument, was unwilling to compromise but rather took turns getting his/her own way with a vengeance, never took the initiative, or had no ambition, etc. These realizations provide the therapist with a helpful corrective to each partner's belief that the other is no longer the person they married and the cause of the marital problems.

Another aid to maintain compassionate neutrality is appreciating the covert, unconscious "deals" that couples make with each other before they marry. For example, the self-involved husband who was attracted to his wife's constricted sense of entitlement can't understand why she is upset when he repeatedly calls to say he will be three hours late to dinner. The long-suffering wife who was attracted to her husband's sense of boundless possibility now resents his selfishness and insensitivity. It gets worse when she learns he's having an affair. The very attributes that initially attract members of the couple are invariably the ones they complain about when, years later, they seek couple therapy. The therapist who has not yet grasped this dynamic may easily end up blaming one member of the couple for their chronic difficulties.

Another situation where the therapist may lose compassionate neutrality and permanently take sides occurs when it becomes apparent that one member of the couple is having an affair. This disclosure may affect the therapist in several ways. If the therapist happens to be in or has been in a marriage where the partner had an affair, the therapist may over-identify with the cuckolded spouse. Therapists may have strong moral values about infidelity that get displaced onto the therapy. Whatever these values are, they make it difficult not to make judgments that serve to shut down further exploration. The therapist may participate in the cuckolded spouse's demand for details of the affair. Such a stance contributes to the marriage becoming a police state, with the therapist siding with the interrogator spouse. An obsession with finding out *all* the details of the affair creates an atmosphere of unremitting suspicion. Further exploration of the details of the marriage becomes impossible. Such a therapy is better served by a therapist who subscribes to the idea that marital trust means "not having to know everything" combined with exploring the causes of the affair. Without such a stance, the philanderer is seen as ruining the marriage.

And finally, two other factors may obscure the fact that each member is contributing 50% of the marriage's difficulties. One has to do with the suppression of important information. Non-disclosure of misappropriated marital funds may give an incomplete picture of what is taking place in the marriage. The other has to do with unconscious processes such as projection. For example, spouse A's conviction that spouse B is intent on leaving the marriage may turn out to represent the first indication that it is spouse A who is intending to leave the marriage.

I have emphasized the importance of the therapist's overall compassionate neutrality despite the temporary siding with one member of the couple that is inevitable in couple therapy. There is one important exception to this statement: when battering occurs in the marriage.[1] Such a marriage may have started out with each member contributing 50% of the couples chronic difficulties. The battered party—invariably the woman—mistook the hyper-control of her husband for caring and her husband needed someone with low self-esteem to serve as a distraction from attending to his own self-esteem issues. However, once battering occurs and a lethality assessment indicates that (usually) the woman is in grave or mortal danger, the therapist needs to help the woman make plans to ensure her safety. The therapist must be aware that such a necessary step may possibly increase her patient's degree of danger in the near future. A restraining order may be necessary.

Note

1 Bograd, M., & Mederos, F. (1999). Battering and couples therapy: Universal screening and selection of a treatment modality. *Journal of Marital and Family Therapy*, 25: 290–312.

Chapter 7

Internal conflict can masquerade as dialogue.

You are feeling withdrawn, disinterested, in fact, lonely. You have experienced this feeling with this patient before. You are trying hard to listen and suddenly realize that this patient is not hearing what you are saying. He has been talking about the anti-depressant medications he is taking and is confused about their side effects. "Why," the patient wants to know, "should I be getting dry mouth and nausea when I didn't do anything wrong?" Apparently making complete sense to the patient, this comment completely flummoxes his therapist. Hoping to shift the conversation from a moral to a more neutral plane his therapist explains about medication: "Anti-depressants do not know they are anti-depressants; all they 'know' is that they are molecules that have many properties, one of which is to relieve depression. But these particular molecules have other effects and, in your case, happen to cause dry mouth and nausea." Feeling satisfied and secure in the belief that his patient will be reassured by this explanation, instead, a rude surprise awaits the therapist. The patient replies, "But I've tried to be good my whole life. Don't you remember how I was the peacemaker at my mother's second marriage when everyone in my family was so upset?"

What is going on here? Why is there such a disconnect between patient and therapist? The answer to this question is both profound and simple. The therapist proceeds on a mistaken premise, namely, that he and his patient are having a conversation when, in fact, the patient is absorbed in tension between two parts of himself. One part insists that he is a good person, that he has done nothing wrong. The other part of the internal dialogue, which cannot be heard—like a telephone conversation only one side of which is audible—could not disagree more. That part reviles the patient in the most severe terms about all the horrible things the patient has done and, even more devastating, all the ways in which the patient is a horrible person. The accusations are not a one-time occurrence; instead, there is a continuous neural firing, an unrelenting bombardment the summation of which translates somehow into "You are bad."

Guilt is the supreme ruler here and can't be dethroned, its decrees being apparently incontrovertible. As in Kafka's *The Trial*,[1] the patient is guilty of a horrible crime, the nature of which is never specified. The person is simultaneously convinced of his guilt and incessantly asserting his innocence. So persecuted is the

DOI: 10.4324/9781003174608-10

person that at times he even doubts his innocence. Preoccupation with this never-ending, internal, uncivil war saps the person's energy, leaving little available to attend and respond to external reality.

What makes the therapist blind to the patient's self-absorption? Is it a narcissistic issue, namely that the therapist experiences difficulty acknowledging that he is irrelevant to what is transpiring for the patient? Isn't the therapist sufficiently important, his knowledge even more so, that the patient would hang on his every word? Not so. The noxious internal signals command attention, consigning the therapist to irrelevance at worst, or to being no competition at best. Perhaps it is the simple habit of assuming that when two people exchange words, they are actually having a conversation that distracts the therapist from appreciating the patient's self-absorption.

Consider further the patient's predicament. For a simple stimulus, nature has devised a simple solution. Touch a hot radiator, an afferent neuron takes the message directly to the spinal cord where a synapse links it to an efferent neuron that excites a contracting muscle. The hand withdraws immediately, pain is avoided or diminished in a millisecond. But what if the stimulus is continuous and unrelenting? A simple neurological mechanism no longer suffices; a more complex, psychological structure is required.

Freud posited a tripartite structure of the mind: Id, Ego, and Superego.[2] The repository of internalized cultural mores, the Superego can range from benign to reasonable to malignant. In its malignant form, its possessor cannot hide from its constant accusations, criticisms, and judgments. Perhaps the greatest relief that therapy can provide to one so tormented is a softening of the Superego. The therapist's compassionate neutrality, curiosity, and non-judgmental, accepting attitude toward the patient combine to achieve what I like to call the "Jergens Lotion effect." It is indeed impressive to appreciate how long it sometimes takes to achieve such a softening effect.

Note that this Pearl does not involve a comment the therapist might make to his patient. Rather, the realization that an intra-psychic conflict can masquerade as conversation is a reminder to the therapist that serves to inform how he "listens" to his patient's material, what he then says, and how he says it.

An extreme example of this dynamic occurred when I was a liaison psychiatrist in an acute physical rehabilitation hospital. I was asked to consult on a 56-year-old widow with diabetes who had suffered a stroke and appeared quite depressed. During the interview what struck me most was her incredulity that she had suffered a stroke. I told her that I was curious about her disbelief since I assumed that she knew that diabetics were susceptible, among other medical maladies, to having a stroke. She pulled herself up in the bed in protest and responded to my comment by saying, "But doctor, I have taken every precaution." I asked what she meant. She answered, "Doctor, I drank my urine every day." Realizing that this guilt-ridden woman was ensconced in her "uncivil internal war," and not wanting to interrupt her narrative, I said, "And you still suffered the stroke." I took her comment to mean that she had been a good person who didn't deserve such a severe punishment. She appreciated my understanding and kept talking.

Most likely such patients have received ample reassurance from people in their lives that they are not bad people. The therapist's support, though well intentioned, is not empathic; it does not acknowledge the patient's dilemma from the patient's point of view. A more helpful comment, in the form of a question, might be, "Would it be fair to say that you never seem able to get relief from these relentless self-accusations?"

Notes

1 Kafka, F. (1925). *The Trial*. Berlin: Verlag Die Schmiede.
2 Freud, S. (1923–25). *Id, Ego and Superego*. XIX volume of the Standard Edition of the Complete Works.

Chapter 8

One of the fringe benefits of being a therapist is all that we learn from our patients.

There are so many ways that my patients have contributed to my ongoing education. The privilege of seeing up close how patients decide to live their lives provides the opportunity to reflect on and put into perspective what is important in life. Some patients inspire. Despite their struggles with anxiety and depression, they contribute to their communities, give to charity, and educate themselves about the important issues of the day. Some of our patients deal impressively with existential issues such as aloneness, finding meaning in their lives, coping with falling ill, and dying. We wonder whether and hope that we will be able to do as well. Other patients lead such hurried lives that their blessings are unable to overtake them. They provide an opportunity to take a hard look at our appointment book and ask, "Do I really need to schedule 45 patient hours/week? How do I feel as I listen to a patient's account of her daughter's soccer game when I can't find time to attend my own child's school play?" Sometimes our patients help us as much as we help them.

During my first year of psychiatric residency, each resident was assigned one chronic patient at a state hospital in the city. My patient, Sophie, was a woman in her fifties who had the diagnosis of simple schizophrenia. One day she asked me, "Doctor, how do I know when I'm done wiping off the table?" The question took my breath away. It had never occurred to me before that a person could struggle with such a basic task. Thinking further about the question, I realized that there was more to the question than my patient had probably intended. So many life tasks are never finished. There is always more to be done in maintaining friendships, in learning one's craft, or in the act of self-reflection. What I took away is the realization that every encounter with another person is a potential learning experience.

Occasionally patients' avocations coincide with one's own and become particularly instructive. Carl helped me with my tennis game, but his unwitting instruction had nothing to do with strategy or hitting the ball correctly. He had developed the art of taking the joy out of the game. It was painful to listen to his need to win at all costs rather than working on improving his strokes or enjoying competition. He never felt he was beaten by his opponent's excellent play, only by his own ineptitude. He could never say to his opponent, "Good shot." He described how he

DOI: 10.4324/9781003174608-11

would excoriate himself in matches that he lost: "You suck. Why don't you give up the game?" What better blueprint for how NOT to play the game could I ask for? I would think of Carl when I wasn't playing well. His example has helped me remember to feel grateful for how fortunate I am to still be playing a decent game into my ninth decade.

Other patients, in describing their experiences, deepen our understanding of the degree to which human beings can suffer. A group patient, Denise, whose mother was obsessed with cleanliness, lived in constant fear of her mother's constant criticism. No matter how hard she tried she could never be good enough. In a state of desperation, at three o'clock one morning she lay down on the kitchen floor and poured ketchup all over herself. She hoped that her mother would find her "bleeding" and finally care about and love her. Predictably, that didn't happen. Her mother yelled at her for making a mess. I'll never forget the humanizing effect that her story had on a schizoid man in the group. He said it was the first time he had cried in over 40 years. The haunting image of her lying on the kitchen floor has provided me with a lasting appreciation of human suffering and its countless manifestations.

Some of my patients have provided me with hope about the human condition. Many emerged from early lives with crippling issues that would take a lifetime to resolve—and yet they have persevered. Emily casually told me about an experience in her previous therapy that apparently held no special significance for her. One day when she was too sick to attend a therapy session, she sent a friend in her place. Her father ran the family like a military installation in which she and her three sisters felt like interchangeable members. She worked hard in therapy to rebuild a devastated sense of self. Mark spent his childhood trying to get his narcissistic mother's attention. He became a very successful newspaper reporter at a young age. When he called his mother—who had been named Mother of the Year in Iowa—to tell her that he had won the Pulitzer Prize for reporting, his mother responded, "That's not the Nobel Prize is it?" Though well into his fifties, he was finally able to marry. Trudy came to this country from a small Austrian town as an au pair when she was 18. Within 2 years she married an abusive alcoholic. In therapy she recovered the memory of having been raped at age 15 by a young man in her hometown. She had been naïve about sex at the time. She earned the respect of her therapy group as they watched her change from a victim to a person with a sense of agency. She was able to leave her abusive marriage and earn a degree in library science.

Running psychotherapy groups taught me the importance of recognizing my group members' unrecognized acts of courage.[1] Even the healthiest of us needs to be noticed and appreciated when we have succeeded at accomplishing something difficult. The absence of recognition can reinforce feelings of invisibility, self-doubt, loneliness, unfairness, resentment, and demoralization. Patients have told me that it means a great deal to them when I have recognized their acts of courage, especially when these behaviors have gone unnoticed by the other group members. My understanding of the fear that they have had to overcome to risk these behaviors is what they value the most. Here are a few examples. Nick feels he is toxic to other people. Over time he comes to care about the people in his group. Even though he fears that his very presence could be injurious to those he now cares about, he decides to continue to attend. Alex has used frenetic performance and achievement in unsuccessful attempts to secure love. He decides to be relatively silent in the group to see if he can be accepted for himself rather than for his accomplishments. Frank grew up with a tyrannical, abusive father. Full of dread, he decides to confront a bully who has been taunting another group member. Sam's parents were duplicitous, saying one thing but meaning another. Sam decides to risk asking group members if they harbor thoughts that are at odds with the positive comments they openly express. Borrowing from what I have learned in running groups, I have made it a point in my outside life to recognize and comment on the courageous acts of others.

Patients have also educated me about many of life's paradoxes and enigmas. Some of my healthiest patients came from very difficult backgrounds. Others taught me that there is no necessary correlation between health and success. One philanthropist and corporate board member went into an emotional free fall whenever his elderly mother criticized him. And yet he always looked unflappable. A patient in his late 30s taught me how one comment from a valued other can apparently make a big difference in one's life. He described how as a teenager he was in the outfield shagging fly balls. After making a sensational catch, his cousin yelled out, "You're a natural." The patient concluded from that tribute that because he was a natural, he never had to work hard at anything. He spoke with sadness about feeling like a failure. A devoted couple, married for 15 years, collaborated extremely well in the care of their son who had a major disability. Suddenly and mysteriously, the husband became convinced that his wife was having an affair. He said he would have to leave the marriage if she didn't apologize. His wife said that she couldn't admit to something she wasn't doing. Family and friends were completely shocked by the disintegration of their seemingly model marriage.

Being intimately involved in our patients' lives provides us with lessons for life, opportunities for self-reflection, an appreciation for human suffering and resilience, and a unique exposure to life's paradoxes and apparent mysteries.

Note

1 Gans, J. S. (2005). A plea for greater recognition of our group members' courage. *Int J of Group Psychother*, 55: 575–593.

Chapter 9

Seemingly innocuous patient comments often yield valuable information about the patient, the patient–therapist relationship, and the phase of therapy.

Experience has shown that material with which patients start and end sessions often has more significance than initially assumed. The patient has an almost infinite number of topics to select from to start the session; exploration of why the patient selected the material she did frequently contributes to a deeper understanding of the patient. A neurologist, in having a patient stand on one leg with his eyes closed, can infer much about the patient's overall neurological status. In a similar way, a therapist exploring a seemingly casual remark at the beginning or end of a session secures information about the nature of the transference and countertransference, the state of the alliance, unconscious material striving for consciousness, and the phase of therapy—or even something that took place just prior to the appointment. My discussion will limit itself to one particular topic that usually receives attention at the beginning of a session, namely a patient's lateness.

The patient who comes late to a therapy session has a number of options. She can explain why she is late. If she does address why she is late, her explanation could have a particular tone: apologetic, frantic, angry, sad, disappointed, or indifferent. She can begin the session with no explanation for why she is late. She could respond to what she senses her therapist's reaction is to her lateness.

If a patient comes late to a session and immediately explains that that she was caught in an unavoidable traffic jam, the statement could have a variety of meanings. These various meanings would depend on the phase of therapy, the nature of the transference, the state of the alliance, the developmental level of the patient, the patient's default position, the therapist's attention to the framework of therapy, and a host of contextual factors. If the explanation is a one-time occurrence rather than the result of a pattern, it probably is best left unaddressed.

Upon learning that the patient's lateness was due to traffic, there are a number of possibilities that the therapist might consider. Had there been a forecast of heavy snow for that day and had the patient planned accordingly? Does the patient frequently cite bad traffic as the reason for being late? Is the patient more annoyed or angry with the unpredictable traffic or more concerned about having missed out on therapy time?

Aside from these considerations, the therapist could wonder, "What does she want to convey in telling me this information?" Is it simply the common courtesy

DOI: 10.4324/9781003174608-12

that one would extend in a friendship? If the therapy is in the early stage when the patient does not yet fully appreciate the differences between friendship and a therapeutic relationship, her comment makes sense. In friendship, it is common courtesy to explain one's lateness as a way of indicating that you appreciate that the other person's time is valuable and that the other person has made the effort to be on time (assuming that was the case). In therapy, on the other hand, especially as it progresses, rituals such as explaining lateness are grist for the therapeutic mill. By the second year of therapy, the patient could well expect that her therapist might inquire why she is volunteering an explanation of her lateness.

There are several possible explanations. One might be that the patient still doesn't appreciate the difference between therapy and friendship. Is this lack of understanding due to the fact that the therapist conducts therapy with a there-and-then focus and does not invite his patient to look inward? Or, has the therapist encouraged introspection and the patient, so far, has shown a limited capacity or inclination for it? Another possibility might be that she wants to reassure her therapist that she is serious about her therapy, that she doesn't take being late lightly. If such a thought has never crossed the therapist's mind—namely, that his patient doesn't take her therapy seriously—the therapist might inquire further about the patient's reason for providing the information. Maybe the explanation is as simple as the fact that the patient is self-conscious about recent missed sessions due to illness and job responsibilities. Or does the comment indicate something more significant that the patient is only faintly becoming aware of: an objection to dealing with emerging shameful material—or even a wish to leave the therapy?

The comment about the traffic may have an apologetic as opposed to an informational flavor, and a familiar one at that. The patient has regaled her therapist with one story after another about how nothing she does for her husband is ever good enough, about how he relentlessly finds fault with everything she does. Is the patient expecting or inviting her therapist to scold her for being late and pre-empting such criticism with an explanation? Perhaps the patient has already been successful in getting her therapist to be annoyed with her lateness, an unusual reaction for her therapist. An exploration of the patient's expectation can result in a corrective emotional experience as the patient realizes that her therapist is simply curious about, and not critical of, her lateness.

If the tone is apologetic, other meanings may be involved. Since in being late the patient is losing out on time for her therapy, why would she want to lose even more time by apologizing? Is it possible that the patient still experiences the therapy as belonging more to her therapist than to her? Translated, her explanation about the traffic could be taken to mean, "I apologize for wasting *your precious time*." It has been my experience that patients value their therapy time in proportion to how far they have come in valuing themselves. What does that mean exactly? They have come to appreciate that their feelings, their fantasies, their thoughts, their associations, and their bodily states all have importance. They have come to realize that it is in working on their thoughts, feelings, and fantasies toward their therapists that they do their deepest and most important work. They feel deeply that they have the right to be here, not just in the office, but also on this earth—in short, that they truly matter.

Group therapy captures another dimension: do the members of the group feel they matter to each other? A patient comes late to his therapy group and another member caringly and innocuously inquires, "Why were you late?" The tardy member could react in a variety of ways: feeling cared about, having his privacy invaded ("it's none of your business"), feeling interrogated, disbelieving that the question conveyed caring. The way the person takes the inquiry may be quite revealing. The person who feels cared about demonstrates a healthy openness to the caring of others. The person who feels his privacy has been invaded reveals a fragile self that requires insulation from others. The person who feels interrogated displays a profound distrust of others. The person who doubts the sincerity of others' caring may have a suspicious nature or, in this instance, have reason to doubt such sincerity based on previous group interactions with that member.

How might someone who has done a considerable amount of work in therapy handle being late to a therapy session? Most likely she will not explain why she was late. She understands that her therapist is not looking for an explanation. She realizes that the loss of therapy time is hers and, since she is paying for the time, she is not hurting or inconveniencing her therapist. If her therapist were to inquire about any thoughts or feeling she might have about being late, her likely answer would be disappointment, regret, or a sense of loss.

I have taken the responses that patients make about being late as an example of seemingly innocuous statements that nevertheless can have important significance. Since such responses—or nonresponses—invariably come at the beginning of the session, they take on an additional significance. What seems at first innocuous may prove to be the key to revealing hidden meaning.

Chapter 10

Shame is a painful, ubiquitous, debilitating, and often hidden emotion.

A young couple has been physically intimate for some time, but the man, Scott, is bothered by one aspect of their sexual relationship. Whenever they make love, his girlfriend Lois insists on having the lights turned out. Scott tries to be supportive and encouraging by telling her that she has a beautiful body and that she has nothing to be ashamed of. Finally, Lois says to Scott, "What makes you assume that it is my body that I don't want to be seen?"

Shame is a painful and uncomfortable feeling, sometimes associated with guilt and anger. While people feel guilty about thoughts and feelings they have or things they have done, shame involves a global condemnation of the self and is not limited to just thoughts, feelings, or actions. Shame makes one want to hide, cover up, shrink, and disappear—even from the face of the earth. Shame can cause one to blush, feel warm, lower one's head, and slacken one's posture. The person feeling shame feels inadequate, unworthy, worthless, in a word, "no good." Given that shame extends to the core sense of oneself, it is not surprising that so many words in the English language express some elements of it: humiliated, embarrassed, degraded, diminished, disgraced, dishonored, mortified, and worthless. We can feel ashamed in our own eyes or in the eyes of others. The essence of shame interpersonally is the fear that if the other person really knew us, he or she would want nothing to do with us.

Shame exists on a continuum. Feelings of awkwardness, discomfort, and embarrassment occupy one end of the continuum. Humiliation, mortification, and disgrace occupy the other end. To complicate and intensify matters, one can feel ashamed of feeling shame. People tend to keep their shame secret where it can fester and become even more debilitating.

Enduring shame has its origins early in life as a result of harmful statements made by parents, siblings, or significant others. Some examples of shaming statements include: "You're stupid, you're disgusting, you don't deserve to exist." "You have ruined my life." "I deserved a child better than you." "You'll never find anyone who treats you as well as I do." "My biggest regret in life is having you for a child." "You will never amount to anything." Bullying can leave deep and indelible emotional scars that diminish one's sense of self-worth. Toxic interactions are not confined to words. Physical and sexual abuse and, perhaps even worse, parental neglect, can give rise to feelings of shame and self-loathing.

DOI: 10.4324/9781003174608-13

The deceptive thing about shame is that despite its pervasive negative effects on a person's entire sense of self, *people entering therapy rarely mention as their chief complaint "I feel ashamed."* Rather, shame is a behind-the-scenes emotion that contributes to depression, social isolation and alienation, low self-esteem, addiction, promiscuity, and other self-destructive behaviors. Since shame is embedded in patients' presenting problems but not explicitly complained about, being able to detect its presence becomes clinically important.[1]

Here are a few ways that shame masquerades. Shame-filled people (unconsciously) deal with this debilitating affect by downloading it onto others. They achieve this effect through a disdainful, contemptuous attitude that creates shame in others who, for their own reasons, are willing to take on this feeling.

Perfectionism can reflect a person's attempt to master and neutralize the opposite condition, feeling really bad about oneself. Perfectionists don't merely want to do very well, they have to; being perfect is a compulsion. A variant of perfectionism is assuming the moral high ground. Here, the virtuous one sucks everything positive into themselves, leaving everyone else feeling inferior.

Envy is another derivative of shame. Envious people covet in others what they feel they lack. Their relentless pursuit of what (they think) others possess insulates them from feeling their own shame.

Men more than women seem to resort to reaction formation in dealing with shame. Men have been socialized to be strong, independent, and action oriented. They often have trouble knowing and accessing what they feel and putting what they feel into words. When they feel weak, they act strong. When they feel ashamed, they act proud. Women who feel an inner sense of unworthiness attempt to counter or neutralize these feelings by compulsively taking care of others whom they consider more worthy.

Malignant messages from early caretakers get internalized as introjects that feel inescapable. You can run away from home but introjects are inside of you wherever you go. Benign stimuli that are misperceived or misinterpreted activate these introjects. The resulting shame feels endless and inescapable.

Treatment of adult behaviors that generate shame have a better prognosis than the treatment of deep-seated childhood shame. For example, shame can result from behaviors such as infidelity, disloyalty, stealing, or betraying confidences that are at odds with one's values and self-image. Such conditions often respond to treatment.

It is also important to note that shame can exert a positive regulatory function. Shame keeps us from participating in behaviors that go against our values and (positive) self-image. We don't cheat on our taxes, park in disabled parking spots, or cut in line in the grocery store. We characterize as shameless people who consistently violate such boundaries.

Many of the chapters in this book describe efforts to make the therapy hour a sacred space where, sometimes for the first time, patients feel safe and trusting enough to talk about shame.

The therapy of a deeply shame-ridden person is an arduous but rewarding long-term enterprise not for the faint of heart. What follows is a description of a two-phase, multi-decade treatment of Anne. There was no problem identifying shame in her case as it permeated every cell in her body.

Phase I of Anne's treatment took place early in my career when I didn't appreciate how my analytic stance worsened her deep-seated sense of shame. Some of my comments required a degree of introspection of which she was incapable. She experienced my not being omniscient or omnipotent as signs of her worthlessness. It was difficult for her to understand that she wasn't responsible for other people's imperfections. She felt my interpretations were sadistic. "You're sitting there with a cattle prod in your hands getting pleasure from the pain you're causing." The treatment was too depriving and only served to confirm in her mind her pervasive sense of badness. At the same time, she became aware of the huge amount of hate and resentment she carried around and had a relationship with a therapist whose caring for her was not diminished by those feelings. She attended sessions faithfully and was always on time. She paid her bill in a timely fashion. She left therapy after 9 years in treatment.

Sixteen years later she returned to therapy when she saw me quoted in the newspaper about the murder of someone who lived across the street from me. She was worried that I might not be OK after the neighborhood tragedy. She was moved and incredulous to learn that I had wondered over the years about how she had been doing. Over those 16 years she continued working as a manager for a family business and made new relationships. She joined and held the positions of secretary and treasurer in an animal rights organization. There she met and began living with Sam, a financially successful engineer. They spent many enjoyable weekends on his 35-foot sailboat and went on many luxury cruises. There was no sexual component to their relationship.

As phase II of therapy commenced, and after having matured somewhat as a therapist, I recognized that my previous approach had not considered the extent of her fragility and her deep sense of worthlessness. As I was to learn, her significant progress in the intervening 16 years had done little to modify her basic feelings of shame and self-loathing.

I changed my approach and saw that she benefited from conversation, kindness, support, and my ability to contain her self-hatred and periodic disappointment in me. As I began to appreciate her daily suffering, I became much more accepting of her profound deficits. I extended hope that she couldn't generate for herself.

I realized that I couldn't make up for the neglect and abuse of her early years but there were things I could do to be helpful—even if I still imagined that some of my early supervisors might disapprove. When I was on vacation, I would send her a postcard. I allowed her to take a photograph of me that provided comfort when I was away from the office. I told her jokes and, at her request, the same one over and over. She experienced the repeated telling of that joke as if it were a lullaby. I refused the hugs she requested at the session's end, telling her that I thought my doing that would be overly stimulating and too confusing for her. As a solution, I did allow us to touch index fingers at the end of a session, which seemed to lessen her feeling of being an "untouchable." We learned that we both raised dahlias and over the winter I let her store my dahlia tubers in her basement. At her request she took home over the winter one of my office plants that she thought wasn't thriving. She thought of taking care of my plant as reparation for my having to suffer being with such a worthless person. I reframed her caring for the plant as something good and life affirming about her. I gave her credit for her compassion for animals and the care she lavished on her three cats. I suggested that we continue to talk about any thoughts or feelings she might be having about any of the frame altering behaviors. It is noteworthy that she always respected and never crossed boundaries. She realized that in modifying the frame of therapy I was trying to provide the caring and appreciation that she craved and needed.

I told her that I thought of the therapy as a process in which I was trying to apply Jergens Lotion to her incredibly harsh and punitive superego. Before going on one vacation, I gave her a bottle of Jergens Lotion, which served the function of a transitional object. At her request, I would bring her brochures from conferences where I had made presentations. Although she had to overcome her feeling that she was bothering me, she would call my answering service just to hear my voice. On several occasions she told me that this session would be her last. I would explore with her what it would be like for her to leave therapy—or stay. Usually over the next few days she would phone me to say that she was glad that I was still her doctor and relieved that I did not agree with her transient wish to end the therapy.

Despite this hard work on both our parts over the next 18 years, Anne continued to feel that she was a bad person whom I (or anyone else) would wish to be rid of. Most of the time she felt toxic, broken, and unfixable. She still felt everything was her fault and that she had no right to be on this earth. She said that she still had no idea of what it was like to be a person or be in a relationship. When I would question that appraisal by referring to our relationship, she would say that it felt fake even though some part of her knew it wasn't. On the other hand, when she considered the possibility that my caring—over 27 years—could be real, she would revile herself for being so stupid as to believe that her feelings or mine could be real. I continued to give her credit for the courage it took for her to get through every day. My occasional suggestion that she was afraid to feel any better lest I would suggest that she no longer needed therapy had little effect.

Ten years into phase II, Sam suddenly and unexpectedly asked her to marry him. They had been living together for almost 25 years. Ten years older than Anne who was now 70, Sam was beginning to have serious medical problems. We discussed the pros and cons of Anne's decision. When she finally decided to marry Sam, she asked if I would officiate at the wedding. (In Massachusetts one can get a 24-hour license to perform marriages.) I worried about appearing in an article in the Boston Globe in which I would be portrayed as a boundary violator. I discussed the decision in peer supervision. Despite my concerns, I performed the ceremony that Anne felt was one of most meaningful experiences of her life. The experience was a memorable and important personal and professional experience for me as well. Anne invited my wife and me to attend the reception and dinner. Anne accepted my explanation of why I thought it best that I confine my participation in the wedding to officiating.

After five years of marriage, Sam had several life-threatening medical events. If it were not for Anne's heroic measures, he would have died after a few of them. I gave her credit for her caring and devotion. She then developed a chronic neurological condition and slowly drifted into dementia. Her friend who her drove her to the appointments during her sad decline said that they were the highlight of her week. I visited her a day before she died in a hospice unit.

I have written in such detail about my work with Anne for two reasons. I wanted to let the extent of our work together speak for itself. I also to wanted to make it clear that deep shame originating in childhood often results in mental illness as serious and debilitating as bipolar disorder, schizophrenia, major depression, and chronic anxiety. It was a privilege and deep learning experience for me to get a hard look at the devastating effects of shame in a 27-year treatment over a 44-year period.

Note

1 Gans, J. S., & Weber, R. L. (2000). The detection of shame in group psychotherapy. *Int J of Group Psychother*, 50: 381–396.

Chapter 11

Ideas are one of the most powerful medications.

It is not surprising, given the approximately 16 billion cortical neurons in the average adult cortex, that our ideas develop along circuitous routes in sometimes unexpected ways. Let me tell you about one such experience of my own. During my third year of psychiatric residency, working on a cardiac care unit as a liaison psychiatrist, I performed what turned out to be a memorable experience—most likely more for me than for the patient, a 55-year-old nurse. I learned that before her heart attack, she had been passed over for a promotion. Angry and disgruntled, she planned to hand in her resignation as soon as she was able to return to work.

The idea of her resignation must have percolated in my brain for at least a decade although I don't remember giving it a lot of thought. Years later I recalled the consultation with the nurse. I remembered the detached manner in which she mentioned her intention to hand in her resignation as well the feelings that generated her plan. The resignation letter itself carried so many emotions. In addition to her feeling embittered about being passed over for a promotion, she was envious of her co-workers, resentful over life-long financial constraints, and, most important, never felt appreciated by her mother.

Somehow those 16 billion neurons led me to consider a tangentially related professional behavior of my own, namely, prescription writing. Up to that point I had treated prescription writing as routine. It consisted simply of writing the name, amount and dosage of the medication, along with instructions for taking it, the number of refills, and whether the generic or brand name was indicated—and, of course, the patient's name and the date.

For the first time I thought more deeply and creatively about medication and the physical prescription itself. What came to me was how patients often "medicated" themselves with ideas—some of which had therapeutic effects, some of which had "side effects." For example, unrealistically high expectations served to motivate some people while for others such expectations insured disappointment. In what felt like an epiphany, the following thoughts occurred to me: "Wouldn't it be potentially therapeutic to write for a patient a prescription for medication and, at other times, a 'prescription' that consisted only of ideas, suggestions, commands, and recommendations that were germane to and evolving from our psychotherapeutic work? Wouldn't combining important ideas that were being mined in the

DOI: 10.4324/9781003174608-14

therapy with an actual prescription—a powerful symbol for the achievement of health—be both therapeutic and synergistic?" I gave this combination a name, the Concept-Laden Prescription (CLRx).[1] Here are a few examples:

> *You have my permission, and blessing, to take at least one thing for yourself every day. Sig: one bid refill X 1000 No substitution*—written for a patient who was an expert in self-denial.
>
> *Remember, I am not abandoning you, I simply need a vacation. Sig: one qid refill X 500 No substitution*—written for a patient who experienced (my) absence as abandonment.
>
> *You need to let me have limitations without vilifying me. My limitations are no reflection on your worth as a person. Sig: one qd refill X 10,000*—written for a patient who could not tolerate anything less than perfection in her therapist.

I vividly recall the playful delight that patients and I experienced when I would write such a prescription, especially the first time. While the patient was telling his/her story, I would reach for my prescription pad and write out a prescription that spoke to something from which the patient suffered. While I was writing the prescription, the patient continued on with his/her narrative while also (probably) thinking, "What the hell is he doing? Is he even listening to me?" For example, for the patient immobilized with worry, I might write, "Just remember, no news is no news (not bad news). WHY PAY TWICE? If it turns out to be bad news, you and I can deal with it then. Refill x 10,000, no substitution." I would then hand the prescription to the patient. Mild annoyance would quickly turn into an expression of appreciation and a feeling of being thought about and attended to. I might even add, with mock seriousness, "I expect you to carry that with you at all times."

A traditional prescription conjures up the vision of the patient being acted upon by the recommendation of the physician. The CLRx suggests collaboration between doctor and patient: "Here is an idea that has evolved from the work between us—let us see what more *we* can learn and consolidate about it."

The use of ideas rather than pills enables the therapist to make suggestions that can help the patient actualize behaviors that, previously, were difficult to accomplish. Consider the following case example: A woman in her 40s with many admirable qualities reported that after telephone calls with her highly critical mother, she would feel defenseless and would go into a free fall that would last for days. Although a sustained inquiry into the dynamics of this interaction resulted in the patient's awareness that she had become an unwitting receptacle for her mother's projected low self-esteem, she continued to be devastated by these conversations. I wrote her the following CLRx with the instruction that she keep it by her telephone: "Mother, what do you think it is about YOU that makes it so difficult for YOU to appreciate me?"

The CLRx provided my patient the opportunity to speak the formerly unspeakable, to think about why doing so was so difficult, and to experience what it felt like to risk such a behavior. The CLRx also provided the occasion to revisit the transference and see whether there were any things that my patient was currently finding it difficult to say to me.

I wrote CLRx prescriptions for the most part in the working through phase of therapy after the patient had already "suffered" the truth of certain insights and was in agreement with them. Patients had usually been in therapy for at least 2 years before I wrote them a CLRx. Typically, these patients, who made up 10%–15% of my patient roster, had serious pre-oedipal difficulties involving such basic matters as their right to exist, profound distrust, conviction of their badness, invalidation of their feelings, compulsive need to perform good deeds to obtain love, and a precarious sense of self. I might not write a CLRx for a couple of years and then write 3 in 1 year, depending on newly arising insights that I thought could be consolidated with behavioral recommendations. I found that the CLRxs tended to solidify understanding when the therapeutic alliance was strong and resistance was low.

A major aim in writing a CLRx is to relocate and expand therapy to a different space that allows for greater spontaneity, playfulness, and creativity. Since no two clinical situations are the same, the therapist's introduction of the CLRx should be dictated by the needs of the patient, the phase of the therapy, and the state of the transference, countertransference, and the therapeutic alliance. Occasionally, I would use the CLRx to suggest a book, usually a novel or short story, the discussion of which I believe would illuminate a current issue in the therapy. Kafka's "Metamorphosis" is an example of such a literary recommendation.[2]

It has been my experience that the effectiveness of the CLRx derives from both the writing of the message and the medium on which it is written. The therapist takes the time and effort to put into writing on a prescription form an important idea that the therapy has yielded. This unexpected and unusual activity can reflect a caring that the patient has unconsciously come to expect *without actually appreciating*. As Benjamin[3] has pointed out in her writings on intersubjectivity, therapy involves the *recognition* as well as internalization of the (m)other and, in this instance, the therapist. The concrete nature of the CLRx makes it more difficult for patients to take their therapists for granted. The idea, "You think about me and care about me" becomes more real. Several of my patients have been carrying CLRxs in their wallets and purses for more than 20 years!

Since many of the clinicians reading this book will not be psychiatrists, how is the CLRx relevant to them? My answer is not to let reality get in the way of therapeutic possibility. One can always say to the patient, "If I were a doctor and could write you a prescription, here is what I would write." In lieu of a prescription form, the non-psychiatric therapist could use his/her professional stationery. Ordinary language could replace medical jargon; take the pills 4 times/day rather than qid. Some patients would get in the swing of the creative exercise and others wouldn't. Those reactions might serve diagnostic as well as therapeutic purposes.

If there is any doubt about the power of ideas in human affairs, one need not look any further than our present political scene. Some people are fervent about the idea that not wearing a mask in the time of COVID-19 is an expression of their political freedom. They are willing to die for this idea. On the other side, people are adamant that wearing a mask is responsible behavior and shows concern for other people as well as oneself.

What is relevant to psychotherapy in this discussion is that these differing ideas about mask wearing are powered by strong underlying feelings. Similarly, the behaviors that the CLRx recommends address powerful feelings that have compromised patients' lives, and feelings like shame, guilt, low self-esteem, self-effacement, and self-loathing.

The psychodynamic approach usually focuses on thoughts, feelings, fantasies, conflicts, inhibitions, and wishes associated with a behavior. I seldom focus on behavior alone, and yet the CLRx addresses and promotes behavioral change. The unusual importance that the CLRx places on behavior would usually catch my patients' attention—perhaps capitalizing on the element of surprise. They took the recommendation to heart because, clearly, I thought it was important enough to write it on a prescription form. If or when patients inquired about this highly unusual emphasis, I said that I thought the behavioral recommendation in the CLRx would help consolidate insights that the therapy had produced.

Because the CLRx is a novel use of a prescription form, it can open up for discussion the whole topic of medication, including how prescribing medication affects the dynamics of the therapist/prescriber-patient relationship. This area of inquiry is especially important in the present when biologic psychiatry is in ascendance. Patients today, more than ever, tend to believe that their psychiatrists are highly invested in the effectiveness of the drugs they prescribe. Sensitive to this attitude, patients may be more reluctant than they realize to tell their psychiatrists that the drugs are not helping them. Certain patients may be more concerned about disappointing their therapist-prescribers than about pursuing their own welfare. So many questions—often shared by psychiatrist and patient alike—never get broached and discussed: "What is actually helping me in this therapy, if anything at all? Is it the medicine? Is it the knowledge, comments of the therapist? Is it our hard work together? Would I have made progress or be the same without the medication or the therapy?"

Patients need therapists who can discuss these questions honestly, who can overcome self-interest in the service of pursuing the truth (with a small *t*). A therapist's decision to take a time-honored symbol to suggest the potency of ideas (as well as pills) has a way of dethroning the majesty of medication. It is unlikely that a true believer in medication's effectiveness would behave in such a manner. Similarly, the same therapist would not deify therapy to the exclusion of medication when its use was indicated. What patients find therapeutic is their therapists' dedication to pursuing an even-handed discussion rather than promoting their "product," be it medication or therapy or both.

By creatively validating ideas and their power in psychotherapy, the therapist's use of the CLRx can contribute to the following therapeutic aims:

- replacement of passivity with the opportunity for more active collaboration in, and responsibility for, the therapeutic process;

- relocation of therapy to a different space that allows for greater spontaneity, playfulness, and creativity and less risk of judgment and disapproval;
- receptivity to an authentic exploration of the value of medication, be it molecular or ideational, in the therapeutic process;
- enhanced trust in therapists who put unbiased exploration ahead of self-interest;
- increased effectiveness of therapy by adding a behavioral dimension to a psychodynamic approach.

Notes

1 Gans, J. S. (2006). The Concept-Laden Prescription. *Psychiatric Times*: 16–17.
2 Gans, J. S. (1998). Narrative lessons for the psychotherapist: Kafka's "Metamorphosis." *American J of Psychother*, 52: 352–366.
3 Benjamin, J. (1995). *Like Subjects, Love Objects*. New Haven, CT: Yale University Press.

Part III

Clinical Pearls

Chapter 12

Shifting focus from there-and-then to here-and-now

"That is very interesting but unfortunately it is not therapy."

Molly spends one session talking exclusively about her boss's narcissism, micromanaging style, and her office mate's obsequious catering to the boss's every whim. The next session she speaks about her landlord's failure to maintain the property. On another occasion she faults the city's public transportation system. Nothing she talks about indicates internal reflection or attention to her relationship with her therapist. Perhaps, her therapist hypothesizes, Molly requires some additional psycho-education about the therapeutic process. Further explanations about the therapist's and the patient's tasks in the therapeutic enterprise do not help. She continues her litany of complaints from session to session. Perhaps Molly's main issue is trust and she needs to protect herself with a seemingly endless store of grievances. Hopefully patience, understanding, empathy, and the passage of time will yield a more workable patient. Such proves not to be the case. Molly, it appears, is a "chronic complainer."[1] The therapist's task is to see if there is a way to help her become uncomfortable with this form of self-protection and style of relating to others, to make the ego-syntonic ego-dystonic. Her therapist attempts to accomplish this goal with a here-and-now comment said to Molly with compassionate seriousness "That"—her complaint of the day—"is very interesting but unfortunately it is not therapy."

Frank's style of relating illustrates a more virulent but similar challenge to the therapist. Unlike Molly's therapy, Frank's 6-session therapy was brief—2 3-session treatments separated by 4 months. In addition to having little to no understanding of what therapy is about and even less interest in finding out, Frank "introduces" himself through intimidation.

Frank is physically imposing and immediately in the first session expressed anger that the magazines in the waiting room are out of date. He stated that he expected the magazines to be up-to-date when he returned for the next session. While the comment seems trivial, the emotional experience did not. I experienced a real threat in his expectation/demand and felt frightened. I realized that if and until I am able to deal with the intimidating way he introduces himself, all else that takes place would be pseudo-therapy. As he tells his story, I think about how I might address his intimidation.

DOI: 10.4324/9781003174608-16

Frank is a 42-year-old married father of girls 14 and 10. He suffered a disability when a tree he was taking down fell and shattered his leg. His insurance company was giving him a hard time about his disability status, and he was depressed by role reversal at home as his wife was now the only breadwinner. His physical therapist became concerned that Frank's escalating anger was a threat to his children's safety and referred him for psychotherapy. The threatening way Frank introduced himself helped me understand his physical therapist's concern. Although Frank was not psychologically minded, he was concerned enough about his barely contained anger and his children's welfare that he followed up on his referral to therapy. I tried to form an alliance with him about all the things in his life that felt out of control. Despite these attempts, Frank seemed resentful that he *had* to see me in therapy, as if I was making him attend the sessions. He conveyed the sense that, since he was paying me, it was my job to fix him and, given that that was my job, why wasn't I doing it—*now*.

Frank came to 3 therapy sessions and then abruptly stopped. He did not respond to a follow-up letter I sent him regarding his intentions regarding therapy. Four months later he re-contacted me and wanted to be seen immediately as his situation had deteriorated. His wife had recently asked for a divorce, his insurance company was still jerking him around, and he was now living in his sister's basement apartment where he was afraid of her German Shepherd.

In his fourth session after a 3-month hiatus, Frank resumed bullying me: "The magazines in your waiting room are still out of date." I re-experienced the fear I felt in our first 3 sessions. As Frank described the details of his worsening domestic and vocational situation, I remembered that although his wife's insurance paid several months ago for his 3 sessions, Frank had never paid his 3 3-dollar co-pays. Thirty minutes into the 50-minute session, I decided to interrupt his there-and-then narrative and introduce a here-and-now topic: his unpaid bill. Fastening my metaphorical seatbelt and noticing my quickened pulse rate and sweaty armpits I asked, "I wonder if you have any thoughts about your bill?" Angrily Frank retorted, "Insurance paid your bill, didn't it!" "Yes," but you never paid your co-pay." Leaning forward on the edge of his chair in a threatening manner, Frank fired back, "Are you shitting me? At a time like this you are going to bring up 9 bucks?" "Yes, would you like to know why?" "Yeah, why?" "You have been telling me about all the things in your life you have no control over, your leg injury, how your insurance company has been jerking you around, the role reversal at home, and now the impending divorce. With so many things out of your control, isn't it reassuring that one thing at least is in your control?" "Yeah, what's that?" "You can decide whether or not to pay me your co-payment." A tense silence and a penetrating stare. Finally, "Do you have change for a twenty?"

Notice that in themselves the magazines and the 9 dollars are trivial. What is not trivial are Frank's threats regarding the magazines and my decision to push-back about his casual disregard of his financial responsibility. I am comfortable dealing with the psychodynamics of money but usually wait until a robust therapeutic alliance has developed. In this case, however, I needed to reassure him that

I would not allow myself to be pushed around, an important message to someone worried about harming his children.

After the confrontation, Frank's intimidating presence seemed magically to disappear and I felt more relaxed. I learned about his parent's divorce that occurred when his father was also 42 and his upset over his 14-year-old daughter's burgeoning sexuality and sexual acting-out. It turned out, however, that I was more optimistic about the treatment than I had any right to be. After the 6th session, he again left therapy abruptly—this time for good. He never did pay for those last 3 sessions as he was no longer on his wife's insurance and he never responded to the bills I sent him.

In an ideal therapy, after a time, I would have been able to establish a safe and trusting (enough) relationship with Frank where I could have explored his concerns about his external and internal (emotional) reality and formed an empathic connection with him. I found no opportunity to accomplish those goals because of his intimidating presence, my feeling threatened, and the abrupt way he left the therapy. Three and one-half sessions with Frank reinforced my initial impression that I would have to deal with Frank's intimidation if a meaningful therapy was ever to materialize. I felt the best way to accomplish this possibility was to deal with *our* here-and-now financial reality, despite the discomfort that approach entailed.

Frank introduced himself through intimidation. To ignore this introduction would have been to embark on a pseudo-therapy with a powerful message to the patient: you can count on me to *overlook* the most challenging parts of you. Even though the patient was not interested in or aware of what the work of therapy consists of, he had an experience with a therapist who did not shirk from the emotionally challenging work. Moreover, until the intimidation was dealt with, there was no way of knowing whether Frank actually had the interest or capacity to become a viable patient.

What can get lost though in considering what approach would have been best for Frank is how confronting his intimidating behavior from the start—in this example, in the here-and-now—affects the therapist's professional esteem and competence. It takes courage to take the patient's best shot, not side step it, not criticize, and, with curiosity, welcome his threatening behavior for exploration. While no one else would know, each one of us realizes whether or not we have stepped up to the plate and accepted the challenge. Harder to calculate is the therapist's sense of personal and professional self-esteem and how facing or shrinking from challenges like Frank's intimidating style contributes to that reckoning.

I never said directly to Frank "That is very interesting but unfortunately it is not therapy," but indicated as much by trying to give him a sense of what does constitute therapy. My confronting Frank about his payment behavior was a first step in that direction. In effect I was saying to Frank, "It is fine if you bring your intimidation into the office, be it around my magazines or your payment for therapy—as long as you are able and willing to talk about the feelings involved. Simply indulging that behavior is not therapy."

Molly mistakes news of the week for therapy; hopefully she just needs more time and therapist caring and understanding before she becomes a patient. Frank indulges his tendency to intimidate, but in order to become a patient he would need to show discomfort with his behavior and an interest in working with a therapist to better understand its origins.

"Isn't it fortunate that all the objectionable people reside outside of our group."

Group cohesion is an important factor in the successful functioning of a psychotherapy group. In the *newly* established group that this chapter focuses on, the sharing of stories and similar experiences helps group members develop an affinity for one another. Two members have cocker spaniels. Three nurse-clinicians exchange clinical experiences and form a strong bond. Two computer programmers seem at home speaking the same technical language. Then there are the losses and failures that are an inevitable part of the human condition and with which everyone in the group can identify. They share their pre-group evaluation experience in which every member presumably agreed to the terms of the group contract that address issues of attendance, confidentiality, out-of-group contact, payment, and termination. Despite their apprehension in attending their first meeting, they all heard the group leader's endorsement of group therapy's many growth opportunities in their pre-group evaluations.

After several weeks, it becomes clear to members, usually before it is articulated, that members don't join a therapy group just to recount similar experiences. They come to work on interpersonal problems, conditions marked by anxiety and depression as well as ego-syntonic behaviors problematic to others. While this awareness is taking hold, another process is occurring: group members, who felt bonded in the joining and belonging phase of the group, start to feel uncomfortable. They begin to identify members they don't like, can't relate to, or are frightened by. Sometimes, the distrusted or rejected others have a vague or striking resemblance to family members or friends that have been troublesome in members' early lives. Other group members, as they regress, start to feel like the group itself creates feelings in them that they suffered in their sibling relationships and childhood friendships. They feel excluded, disliked, unable to be themselves, or exposed with no place to hide. They experience tension as they realize that there is no way to say something about another member without making a self-revelation in the process. They begin to wonder if perhaps they have signed up for more than they bargained for.

The group tries to handle its sense of disappointment in a number of ways. Members arrive late or don't call to say they will not be attending that meeting. Others may pay their bill late or suddenly realize that it takes longer to get to the session than they had anticipated. A group member talks enthusiastically about a lecture on behavioral therapy she attended, a possible first and indirect indication that the psychodynamically oriented group she joined is not to her liking. A member abruptly departs for good, evoking envy in some of the others. Members silently struggle with how to deal with their negative feelings toward one another.

Another way of resolving members' growing discomfort is for the group to focus on people outside the group whom they don't like, are currently having problems with, or have been treated unfairly by. One member enters, holding a traffic ticket, furious at the policeman who could have just as easily issued a warning. Several members enthusiastically enter the conversation, telling about similar experiences. A woman describes how her husband plays golf on the weekends and neglects the family. The group then hears about a landlord who hasn't repaired the heating system and a dinner party where the conversation was boring and the food even worse. The group feels a greater solidarity, and hence, an enhanced sense of security, as it commiserates with one another about "the bad people out there".

As the leader takes note of the group's conversation, she silently generates the following hypotheses. Group members are complaining about people in their outside lives because they are as yet unable or unwilling to broach their growing dissatisfaction with some of the members of the group. She considers the not unlikely possibility that there is discontent in the group about her leadership as well. Could she be the negligent landlord who is not providing enough warmth, the hostess who has convened an unproductive get-together, or the policeman who treats people unfairly? The group, she realizes, is at too early a stage in its development for her to suggest these possible covert meanings. She will save such comments for a time in the future when the group is able to work with metaphor and more abstract ways of thinking. Groups at this early stage tend to hear comments on a concrete level. The dinner party is just the dinner party. Attempting to point out material that is still at an unconscious level would most likely result in shaming. She realizes that she needs to make a comment that will speak to the group's ego, not its unconscious. The comment needs to be both sufficiently benign and yet have enough of an edge to promote group work. When the time seems right, she says, "Isn't it fortunate that all the objectionable people reside outside our group."

What do I mean when I say "when the time seems right"? The leader's process is a combination of cognitive assessment and visceral feel. Group sessions exist in a dialectic tension. The sense of security that results from a feeling of similarity alternates with the tension and conflict that attend risk taking. An impatience with an excessive degree of security—where little psychotherapeutic work is accomplished—leads to a receptivity to dealing with built-up tension and conflict that once dealt with and resolved leads back to a wish for security.

Deciding when the group is ready to forsake security is by no means an exact science. Here are a few considerations I have found helpful in making this decision. Yvonne Agazarian advises group therapists to point out similarities when fractiousness dominates group transactions.[2] She advises group therapists to look for difference when there is an extended focus on similarity. It is when the group becomes impatient with an excessive focus on similarity—and the leader *feels* this to be the case—that the group is most receptive to reflecting on a statement like "Isn't it fortunate that all the displeasing people reside outside our group?"

The group might react in a number of ways to such a comment by their leader. The group may not understand the significance of the comment or they may simply ignore it. And yet, a sustained focus on there-and-then complaints results in understandable dissatisfaction with a group leader who has allowed the group to degenerate into a gripe session where no meaningful therapeutic work is taking place. At that point, somebody recalls a version of the group leader's comment and redirects the group's attention to what is transpiring in the group.

The group leader braces herself at this juncture as she realizes the importance of her becoming a lightning rod for the group's pent-up negative feelings. She knows from experience that the successful processing of these feelings invariably leads group members to become more direct and honest with each other. Group members get a chance to vent their dissatisfactions as the group leader listens with curiosity, understanding, and non-judgment. Empathizing with the disappointment that underlies the anger softens the group atmosphere. Members become reassured that the leader is strong enough to help the group contain and work with strong feelings. Acknowledging mistakes that she has made along the way and that the group has pointed out adds to the group's feeling of safety. At this point, gently nudging the group toward talking about the here-and-now, the leader might ask, "What are people presently afraid of in this group?"

The group eventually takes over the leader's function of directing its attention to the here-and-now. It does so because the work that is accomplished through a here-and-now focus is compelling and speaks for itself. As Willy Sutton said when asked why he robbed banks, "That's where the money is."

In this chapter I've described the thinking and the timing that goes into the leader's redirection of the *new* group's focus from the there-and-then to the here-and-now. Accomplishing this redirection is both challenging and important because it is in the here-and-now that the most important group work takes place. Helping a small crowd of people become a therapeutic entity with an inward focus is difficult to achieve. The comment "Isn't it fortunate that all the objectionable people reside outside of our group" can play an important role in gradually redirecting the group's focus to where its most meaningful therapeutic work will take place.

Notes

1 For more on "chronic complainer," see Chapters 14 and 18.
2 Agazarian, Y. M. (1997). *Systems-centered Therapy for Groups*. New York: Guilford Press.

Chapter 13

Employing irony and paradox for therapeutic purposes

"Could you be a little more *vague*?"

Suppose you grew up in a home with a father who served in the Marine Corps and ran the household like a military operation: morning inspections, required nightly baths, and evening bed checks. Your father made fun of your middle brother who seemed effeminate and who went on to live the tortured life of a closeted gay man. Your youngest brother went to Vietnam, got addicted to drugs, which, 10 years after discharge, led to his untimely, drug-overdosed death. Your mother meant well but as a 1950s housewife did not stand up to her domineering husband, could not countenance divorce, and provided little emotional safety for her sons.

It is usually helpful for the therapist to try to put him/herself in the patient's shoes. Wouldn't it make sense for you to develop camouflage as a survival technique? Blend into the woodwork, don't make waves, and don't confront your father about his treatment of your brother and your mother. You've got a good mind, use it to your advantage in school, and become a better man than your father. It wasn't an approach that anyone suggested; you came upon it naturally, even unconsciously. It worked, you became an architect, married in your early 30s, inherited a step-son, and fathered a child by the time you were 35.

Two major flaws in your personality surfaced gradually in your marriage. First, you had no idea of what you wanted out of your life, what you actually felt, or how important your marriage was to you. The one thing you knew for sure was that you loved to play tennis, a lot of tennis. If you did have other thoughts and feelings about your life experiences or about your wife, you were unable to put those emotions or desires in words. Second, you became an expert at vagueness, a first cousin of camouflage. You never spoke in specifics—which is where feelings reside. You would remember something happening ten times but never what happened one time. You couldn't remember particular examples to buttress your point of view so you were always losing arguments to your wife. You became angry that she was taking 12 years to complete her dissertation but you couldn't feel or express that anger. You felt she never appreciated the slack you took up on the domestic front but, again, you could never express your resentment directly. You played more and more tennis and found consolation in mastering the sport.

DOI: 10.4324/9781003174608-17

You became a competent architect but had difficulty collecting fees. You and your wife began to lead parallel but separate lives that led to her asking for a divorce.

Vagueness confronts the therapist with many challenges. Since working with feelings is our stock-in-trade, patients who provide none in therapy frustrate us. Realizing that our patient is not purposefully being vague tempers our annoyance. We soon realize the patient is totally unaware that he presents himself in this fashion. Learning about the history noted earlier increases our appreciation of the survival value of camouflage, although realizing that vagueness is a derivative of camouflage takes some time.

There is a second reason why we find the patient's vagueness unsettling. As authority figures, the patient expects us, much as he resents us, to have profound insights, definitive answers, and antidotes to complexity. It is tempting to buy into this misconception since, what is equally unsettling, is our awareness of how much we do *not* know. Many a patient locates their intelligence, leadership qualities, and empathic capacity in us. The result is for us to feel unusually competent and for the patient to feel surprisingly depleted, having unwittingly put so much of him/herself in us. The patient's vagueness though reminds us at some basic level of the uncertainty, doubts, and confusions which reside at the core of our comfortable professionalism. If some authority were to ask us to list the exact causes of all mental illnesses, we might seem vague ourselves.

How best to deal therapeutically with vagueness? Since the patient in question happens to have a good sense of humor, and since the culture in which he grew up was stern, regimented and in-your-face, a playful, indirect, approach seems indicated. There can be nothing more comforting to a patient who expects harshness than to find the other non-threatening and relaxed. I remember a patient who dared to share a painful secret: he picked his nose and ate the snot. He thought that doing so, eating his own bodily contents, somehow conferred immunity against disease. In response to this disclosure, his posture indicated a fear of being criticized or shamed. His body noticeably relaxed as he took in my comment: "You mean you give yourself booster shots" to which he replied, "Exactly."

For the patient with the stern, sadistic military father, the question "Could you be more *specific*?" might sound demanding and intimidating. The more playful question, "Do you think you could be a little more *vague*?" finds the patient's comfort zone, an area where he is already an expert. A Cheshire catlike smile probably emerges from one side of my patient's mouth as if to say, "Sure, I would be glad to, I specialize in vagueness." The question "Could you be a little more *vague*?" feigns demandingness, asks the patient to do something familiar while, at the same time, creates mild discomfort by paradoxically inviting the person to enter the foreign territory of specificity. A stern military father would never ask such a question.

"Why is it that I get *deprived* of 50% of your feelings? It doesn't seem fair."

Therapists attempt to create in the therapy hour a distinctive space. We (try to) say things only when it is for the patient's benefit. We privilege process over content. We clarify for patients how therapy differs from friendship: we meet in a particular location, for a set period of time, for a particular purpose and goal, and we charge for our time. We explore comments that would be left unexamined in friendship. For example, we might explore the commonplace expression, "Have a good weekend," said on a regular basis by a patient at the end of her Friday sessions when it is evident that the therapist's weekend is going to be much better than the patient's weekend (as described in Chapter 2).

The comment in the title of this chapter contributes to the same distinctiveness through the use of irony. When someone complains of being deprived of something, that something is usually desirable. "Why didn't I get to taste the cake?" "Why didn't I get a turn?" Or more seriously, "Why was I deprived of my inheritance?"

People tend to think that others are spared, not *deprived* of the less attractive parts of their personality. Someone is feeling deprived of my negative feelings? Come on, you can't be serious! Since when have my hostile, jealous, irreverent, unreasonable, disdainful, demeaning, envious feelings been valued, let alone welcomed? In fact, growing up, many people have suppressed their more mischievous and aggressive parts, complied with parental imperatives in the service of securing love. Think of the behavioral constraints many children grow up with: "Behave yourself," "Be nice to your sister (brother)," "Is that any way to act?" "We expect you to have your homework done before you watch TV." These comments indicate that the child should be good, behave, meet expectations, not make waves, etc. Life is hard enough. Most adults don't need or want more aggravation. Thus, this comment enlarges therapeutic space by indirectly indicating to the patient that many of the ordinary rules and norms of social intercourse don't apply.

The question "Why is it that I get deprived of 50% of your feelings? It doesn't seem fair" is the emotional equivalent of a can opener. It opens up the patient to new possibilities. The patient, it appears, is now free to feel and communicate anything short of physical violence—assuming the patient is willing to work on the material expressed. Despite the therapist's invitation, the patient often remains emotionally constricted. Is it that the patient doesn't understand what the therapist said? Or is it a matter of distrust or disbelief? Whatever the reasons, the question makes it harder for the patient over time to avoid the realization that constraints on emotional expression are coming from within, not from without. The focus of therapy now has a chance to shift from outer to inner, from politeness to authenticity and spontaneity, from being nice to being genuine.

Other approaches, through different methods, also attempt to allow patients a fuller range of emotional expression. Harry Stack Sullivan, for example, spoke about parataxic distortion.[1] In contrast to transference that develops slowly over time, Sullivan thought that the minute the patient and therapist laid eyes on each other, the patient projects onto the therapist (he didn't address the therapist's projections).

How might such a dynamic play out? Let us assume that the therapist is accurate in considering herself to be an interested, caring, curious, empathic helper, and that the patient, on the other hand, is sure that she is a demanding, critical, uncaring, intrusive presence. From the start of therapy, according to Sullivan, the patient experiences the therapist as someone other than the therapist experiences herself to be. As a result, the patient unwittingly preserves as a vital presence an important figure from the past with whom the patient still struggles internally. Since people tend to believe their projections, this altered view of the therapist seems very real and convincing to the patient—and is very difficult to alter.

It is not difficult to appreciate the different feelings the patient would have depending on which view of the therapist is compelling. Believing the therapist to be demanding, critical, uncaring, and intrusive, the patient would most likely feel guarded, suspicious, unsafe, vulnerable, or wary. Most likely, the patient has sought therapy because his misreading of other people—just as he has misread the therapist—is interfering with his satisfactory relationships out in the world.

To be helpful to such a patient, Sullivan contends, the therapist needs to assume a stance that makes it (more) difficult for the patient to maintain such a relatively fixed misperception. Sullivan has named such a stance counterprojective. In assuming a counterprojective attitude, the therapist has to first figure out how she is being misperceived. Is her patient perceiving her as strict or permissive, indulgent or depriving, seductive or aloof, omnipotent or deeply flawed, idealized or cruel?[2]

Let's consider as an example a patient who (the therapist determines) idealizes her. This therapist's inference is based on the fact that her patient never mentions or ascribes any negative motivations to her. For patients who project onto the therapist an idealized, agreeable, extremely benevolent persona, the comment "Why is it that I get deprived of 50% of your feelings? It doesn't seem fair" serves a counterprojective function. If, in reality, the therapist only wanted to hear flattering statements, she would never make such a statement. She is making clear that if the patient has less flattering thoughts and feelings toward her, she's interested in hearing them. The patient's reactions to this statement vary over time. The patient may at first be perplexed, then possibly guarded, then gradually feel reassured that the therapist *really* is interested in all his feelings. This sense of reassurance reduces the patient's anxiety, allowing the therapist to be experienced more as a real person and less as a distorted projection.

If counterprojective statements like the one under consideration serve to illuminate the therapist more as she actually is, they also allow the patient gradually to get in touch with more of his feelings and to feel more secure in expressing them. With more of the patient's feelings in the room, it becomes more difficult for the *therapist to misperceive who the patient actually is*. This is another way of saying that the therapist also needs to work on her misperceptions of the patient. While the counterprojective stance may have clarified the therapist for the patient, the therapist still needs a corrective for her early fantasies of who she imagined the patient to be. To apprehend the reality of the other person is a process that involves psychological work over time. Therapists need to work on their initial perceptions of the patient, some of which—because of the uniqueness of every person's internal world—will inevitably be off the mark. The therapist as well as the patient is at risk of mistaking one part of the person for the whole. Fortunately, there is much more to each of us than that.

Notes

1 Sullivan, H. S. (1954). *The Psychiatric Interview*. New York: W.W. Norton.
2 Havens, L. (1976). *Participant Observation*. New York: Jason Aronson.

Chapter 14

Using countertransference for therapeutic purposes

"I've noticed that almost all of what you've told me is about things outside of you."

Joe and Harry—creators of the Johari Windows—designed a useful way to look at basic human interactions.[1] They created a square with four equal-sized boxes. In box one, the known quadrant, what I know about me, that for example my name is Jerry, is also what you know about me. In box two, the blind quadrant, you know something about me that I don't know about myself; perhaps I'm excessively deferential or sarcastic and don't realize it. In the third quadrant, I know something about me that you don't know about me; for example, I cheat on my income taxes. The fourth, the unknown quadrant, contains all that I don't know about myself that you also don't know about me.

Focus on quadrant two and the dilemma it poses for the therapist: how does a therapist help her patient become aware of blind spots—defenses, mannerisms, self-protective maneuvers. It seems like a contradiction in terms, to become aware of what one doesn't "see." Obviously, there is a time dimension involved.

Mary talks about her relationships at work and is critical of many things: too much socializing by her co-workers; a poorly administered personal savings account; an unreliable landlord who never responds to emergencies; tasteless, over-priced produce at the supermarket. Mary is an unselfconscious grievance collector.

Therapists should be wary of taking away a defense unless they have something better to offer the patient. At the beginning of therapy, they usually don't. The history of the defense, when it started, and what function it has served, is still uncharted territory. By the time a patient shows up in the therapist's office, the solution to a dilemma evolved in childhood, often in the service of survival, is now the very problem that needs attention. For example, Mary thought that the only way to obtain her neglectful mother's care and attention was to complain. As maladaptive as Mary's complaining style may have been, it served some valuable purpose—up until the present. If nothing else, it was there every morning when she woke up, a constant companion in a life possibly devoid of meaningful relationships with others. If Mary is going to consider relinquishing this personality

DOI: 10.4324/9781003174608-18

characteristic, her therapist must help her gradually to become aware of it. Since possessors of annoying mannerisms and maladaptive behaviors are often the last to know about them, helping these patients become more self-aware without shaming them in the process is a real and important challenge. As an initial, hopefully benign, step in this process, I will say to such patients "I've noticed that almost all of what you've told me is about things outside of you." With the wrong patient or flawed timing, even that comment could be heard as critical, not as a simple observation. Therapists should always keep in mind that the effect of their comments might differ sharply from their intent.

While the statement "I've noticed that almost all of what you've told me is about things outside of you" alerts the patient to this fact, it doesn't often follow that the patient soon thereafter starts paying attention to his/her inner life. Rather, some impediment to or impasse in the therapy and an attempt at its resolution can be the turning point in a therapy. Some turning points are as unpredictable as they are inevitable. As the following example illustrates, processing a therapist's gradual development of a perplexing reaction can lead to a therapy more focused on the patient's feelings. Alice rarely spoke of her feelings and instead described at length what transpired in the doctor's office where she worked as an office manager. Alice never missed or was late for a session, made sure that she ended her sessions on time, and apologized excessively if she needed to change an appointment. Alice suffered from severe depression and felt responsible for anything that went wrong. When a series of anti-depressant medications did not help her or caused debilitating side effects—although one eventually did help her—she felt it was her fault. In short, she presented as a very, very good person.

Her therapist began to notice the following pattern in sessions: he would be quite alert for the first 25 minutes but around the half-hour mark would notice that he was becoming extremely tired, hardly able to keep his eyes open. He was proud to report in supervision his valiant efforts to stay awake. It was established in supervision that he was not tired at the beginning of each session but that this pattern had taken hold over the previous month. The supervisor then inquired why the therapist was taking such pains to stay awake when it seemed that his patient was working hard to put him to sleep. The therapist replied that his patient "was such a good person that if he ever fell asleep during the session it would feel like he was driving a stake through her heart." The violent nature of this fantasy seemed to be as lost on the therapist as it would be inconceivable to the patient. The supervisor continued, "If your patient is working this hard to put you to sleep, don't you think it is inconsiderate at best, or sadistic at worst, for you to try so hard to stay awake?"

Shaken by that supervisory question, the therapist decided to let himself feel his sleepiness and make no effort to mask it. After two sessions, the patient screwed up her courage and uncharacteristically asked if he was sleepy. Having had a few weeks to metabolize his countertransference, the therapist was able to answer "Yes" with equanimity. His patient looked devastated. "But, it is interesting," her therapist continued, "I am not sleepy when the sessions begin. Something is going on between the two of us as the session goes on that hopefully we can understand together."

After a prolonged discussion, the following dynamic emerged. Alice realized that she had wanted to talk about something inside of her, something very shameful, which she was finding it very difficult to share. As she tried to distance herself from her feelings, her verbal productions felt lifeless. When she noticed her therapist almost falling asleep, she had the thought, "If he is not interested in me, why should I talk about what I am ashamed of." After this revelation, almost like magic, the therapist felt wide awake, and the patient appeared more animated. Sessions after this one revealed a patient gradually more comfortable with talking about and focusing on her feelings.

This here-and-now interpersonal experience, building on the initial comment that alerted her to her avoidance of her internal life, changed the direction of the therapy. Felt-introspection—at first occasionally about her feelings toward people she worked with and then gradually toward her therapist—began to replace sterile news of the week.

As relational theory has taught us, what transpires in therapy is always co-constructed by the patient and the therapist. Not surprisingly, therapists also bring their blind spots to the healing enterprise. Nothing can motivate a patient to introspect more than a therapist who demonstrates a willingness to do so. The therapist can indirectly indicate such willingness by periodically checking with the patient: "Is there anything I am doing to impede the very process of therapy that I am trying to facilitate?"

"Was the joke I just told for my benefit or the group's benefit?"

Group therapists need to be especially careful in employing humor for several reasons. Humor is a delicate therapeutic tool and, more than other kinds of interventions, its effect can be quite different from what was intended. Such an untoward effect is more common in the early and even middle phases of group therapy when safety and trust are not firmly established and when group members can receive complex communications—like humor—concretely. The group needs time to have confidence in their leader's attunement to their emotional vulnerabilities. The leader needs time to identify those members who have special difficulty in appreciating humor and who are prone to being shamed. There must be time for the group to work through negative transferences and ambivalent feelings toward authority. Once having accomplished those tasks, the group is well positioned to develop a genuine sense of intimacy where the nuances of humor can be worked with productively. The therapist must be realistically confident that he/she possesses qualities necessary for the effective use of humor. These include spontaneity, trust in one's intuitive sensibilities, neutralized aggression, and comfort with self-deprecating humor. Constant awareness and monitoring of countertransference ensures that the humor is for the patient's or group's benefit and not for the therapist's self-indulgence or consolation.

The group leader needs to avoid employing humor in ways that can be either hurtful or harmful. As mentioned, the use of humor early in the group's development is prone to misinterpretation and can be perceived as shaming. A joke that diffuses the constructive exchange of strong feelings, especially shameful or sexual ones, interrupts the development of intimacy. Group therapists who are feeling ineffective might tell a joke to make themselves feel better—and often at a group member's or the group-as-a-whole's expense. Such a blind spot often occurs when a therapist is out of touch with countertransference. And then there are jokes, even ones told in the mature phase of group development, that are driven by unconscious countertransference, as the following example illustrates.

Simone, a single 50-year-old woman, mentioned having recently met Cecil, a man she had dated four times. From what Cecil had told her about himself, Simone thought that he could have been a pedophile, and she learned that his ex-wife had a restraining order on him. After four dates, Simone cut off the relationship. She described as well other things about Cecil that made the leader think she could have been in danger. The group knew how very much she wanted to have a successful relationship and to get married.

At this point I told the joke about the single woman in Florida who lived in a condo and who knew everyone. One day she saw a man at the condo pool who was clearly a newcomer. Striking up a conversation with him she learned that he had been in jail in Pennsylvania for murdering his wife. He had recently been released and had just arrived in Florida. To which information the woman replied, "Oh, so you're single."

The joke did not go down well. The joke is funny because it depicts a woman so desperate to marry that she would consider dating a murderer. Simone was hurt because she didn't consider herself to be desperate, but from hearing the joke, thought that I did. In retrospect, I think the joke resulted from a counter-transference-generated difficulty. Simone had a very difficult father who made her wary of men. I was fond of Simone and, given how hard I had worked with her over many years, I hoped she was feeling closer to me. But when, from time to time, I would check in with her about our relationship, she said nothing had changed. When she mentioned dating Cecil—as I thought about it later—I had unconsciously felt like a spurned lover and the joke was meant to hurt her back. When she asked in the next session why I thought I had done something hurtful, which was unlike me, I explained how I was feeling. She said she appreciated my honesty and it had felt healing. In this example my countertransference was apparent to me in retrospect but not in the moment.

Humor is likely to be effective when the therapist identifies indications for its usefulness. One indication is the promotion of the group's observing ego and self-reflection. Consider a group that is feeling particularly solicitous and positive about a patient, David, who is hypomanic, always has a novel excuse for missing sessions, is contrite about his absences but doesn't change his behavior, and who doesn't let the group know when he will not be attending a session. The group is also aware that David has not returned the leader's concerned emails and phone messages. I was struck by the contrast between my growing irritation at David and the group's predominantly unconditional acceptance of his disruptive behavior. My countertransference awareness led to my being able to employ humor therapeutically.

I disrupted the flow of the conversation and said, "I'm reminded of the policeman who comes upon a man who has just jumped off a bridge in a suicide attempt. The officer throws the man a life preserver and appeals repeatedly and unsuccessfully for the man to grab onto the life preserver. Finally, in a fit of frustration and anger, the cop pulls out his gun and yells, 'Grab onto that life preserver you sonofabitch or I'll fill you full of lead!'" After some laughter, the group began to get in touch with its irritation at the patient. In telling this joke I was concerned that the group would feel that I wasn't concerned about—or was angry at—the patient for his possibly deteriorating condition. Most group members appreciated that the joke was directed at the denial of *their* irritation and was not an indication that I wasn't concerned about David.

Another indication to introduce humor occurred as a result of the group's failure to comment on Ely's persistent idealization of his wife. It was clear that the group was becoming more uncomfortable with these weekly stories that strained credulity. In my countertransference I was feeling embarrassed for Ely because of his glaring blind spot. I decided to tell the story of a parishioner who challenged the minister's contention that Jesus Christ was the most perfect, moral, and loving person who had ever lived. The minister dared anyone in the congregation to cite a person who was as perfect as Jesus. A man in the back of the church said, "I know of such a person." The minister asked incredulously, "Who might that be?" The man answered, "My wife's first husband!" I tried to capitalize on Ely's sense of humor, hoping that at a level of displacement the story would help him begin to think about his faultless version of his wife. Before telling the story, I tried to anticipate the possibility that I might shame him, an outcome that fortunately did not occur.

Isabel created a situation that allowed me to be playful around the fact that with her I could never get anything right. She invariably spoke in the group immediately after I did and would either ignore or refute what I had said. It became clear that we wouldn't be able to agree on which direction the sun set. One day, in the mature phase of group development, I looked at her playfully and asked if she would like to hear about the famous major league pitcher, Lefty. Taken by surprise and looking somewhat confused, she said "Yes." I told her that Lefty was being interviewed by a reporter and asked about his lifetime record of 1 win and 399 losses. The reporter wanted to know how Lefty accounted for his 1 win. Lefty said, "Well, you can't win them all." This joke led to a serious conversation about why this patient needed to have me on the losing end of so many group discussions. I think the joke helped her appreciate that I wasn't taking her oppositionalism personally and, in a playful way, I was curious to learn more about why I never could get anything right with her. Weeks of metabolizing my irritation with her allowed me to make that playful intervention.

Some patients have difficulty accepting positive comments from other group members. Joyce had especial difficulty in that area. One day Bruce complimented her on the mature way she handled a potentially explosive situation in her family. I turned to Joyce and said affectionately, "Are you going to let him talk to you that way?" Joyce seemed to appreciate that the sentence "Are you going to let him talk to you that way" is usually addressed to a person who has been the object of derision. A telling smile crept into Joyce's face as she grasped the irony and felt the affection embedded in my comment.

Sometimes in group therapy difficult situations and feelings arise that the group has either ignored or not found a helpful way to manage. If the time seems right, the leader might intervene with humor, while mindful of the potentially negative effects. Countertransference awareness and monitoring helps the leader avoid humor that is hurtful to a group member or for the leader's, not the group member's, benefit. In this chapter I have illustrated how the leader has employed playfulness and humor as a way to achieve several goals: exaggerate an avoided emotional state to draw attention to it; promote the development of group's observing ego; highlight the group's denial of anger; undercut a member's idealization of his wife; playfully engage a member's negative transference to the leader; and, through the use of irony and mock seriousness, deal with a member's difficulty with accepting praise.

"Tell us one thing about your boyfriend that you *wouldn't* want us to know about."

Human beings are social animals and we care about what other people think of us or of those dear to us. We try to maintain a positive image. We tell white lies to look better than we are. The 3-pound fish we caught becomes a 6-pound fish in the retelling. We develop a narrative that exaggerates our accomplishments. We project our faults and experience them as existing in others. This chapter focuses on another behavior we employ to maintain a positive self- image: omitting certain information.

In one of my groups, Patricia was telling the group about her new boyfriend. The group knew from things she had told us over the 2 years that she had been a group member that she didn't have the best judgment when it came to picking friends, let alone a boyfriend. As she continued to paint a glowing picture of Tom, and because the group seemed to be so pleased for her, I said to Patricia, "Tell us one thing about Tom that you *wouldn't* want us to know."

My comment was aimed at Patricia's internal process: What flaw would she select? How long would it take her to come up with the flaw? Caught off guard by the question before her defenses could mobilize, how would Patricia react to my question? Why didn't she mention the flaw in the first place? Why wouldn't she want us to know about the flaw since none of us is perfect? Or is Tom so perfect that Patricia can't think of even one flaw? And what about the group? At a minimum, what I hoped Patricia and the group would take away from my question was an enhanced appreciation of all the psychic energy that can go into an omission.

I also wondered about the group's responses. In not joining the group's seeming unanimous enthusiasm for Patricia, I thought to myself that the group might view me as the spoilsport, raining on Patricia's parade. I wondered about countertransference reaction and decided to let group process unfold to help me understand what it might mean.

The question served to unearth some of Patricia's basic issues. She came from a home where she could never talk things over with her parents, who were overbearing and intrusive. They were not people she could go to for advice or guidance. Time was never given to choices she was considering so that she had practice considering all the pros and cons of a given decision. Without realizing it, in her 2 years in the group she began to experience the group as if it were her family. Not surprisingly, she had no confidence that the group could be there to help her think objectively about some of Tom's questionable qualities. Furthermore, her emotional core felt too fragile to withstand the many questions the group might ask her about her boyfriend. She was afraid she would either submit to their collective opinion that, interestingly, she imagined would be negative or, while seeming to consider their comments, she would ignore any warning signs that emerged from the group discussion.

Initially, Patricia couldn't think of a flaw to share. Her boyfriend was the youngest of five children, an excellent athlete, and senior class president. While he had been accepted to several excellent colleges, he decided on a lesser one closer to home despite the fact that finances were not a limiting factor. His parents had separated during the spring semester of his senior year in high school and he was worried about his mother, who had been diagnosed with MS during his freshman year in high school. Patricia described him as kind and responsible, and said that he treated her well. They enjoyed hiking and kayaking. She thought they shared similar values. The group thought that Tom was a far better choice than others she had previously mentioned in the group. They wondered, however, whether he would have trouble separating emotionally from home, although they didn't feel this consideration was necessarily a deal breaker. By the end of that session, Patricia was able to admit that she had a similar concern about Tom but was afraid of how negatively she thought the group would respond.

By the end of the session my countertransference reaction became understandable. Patricia had unconsciously trained the group to feel and act like her family. In an effort to be as unlike her family as possible, the group assiduously tried to avoid any hint of criticism. I had somehow internalized Patricia's family's critical reactions and imagined that the group would think critically of me—which they never did—for what was a relatively benign question.

The following week, Patricia told the group that the discussion with them about Tom felt like a corrective emotional experience for her. Subsequently she felt comfortable asking the group for their help when it seemed that she was having difficulty considering their input.

In group therapy it is difficult sometimes to tell whether group members have not noticed certain group phenomena or have noticed but decided not to comment. I have found it to be productive to comment on what I consider to be omissions.

Consider the first group session after my 5-week summer vacation. Out of the 9-member group it was known that 3 would be on vacation when I returned. As members filed into the office and took their seats, the 3 seats next to me—1 to my left and 2 to my right—were empty.

Usually, upon returning from a vacation I would be very happy to see everyone after having been away for so long. (I usually took 3 to 4 weeks off.) Instead of feeling glad to see everyone, I focused on the 3 empty chairs next to me. I noticed my detached and intellectual reaction to the empty chairs and had the following thought: they want to ignore me and hurt me back for taking such a long vacation (and, as I recall, a particularly wonderful vacation). An old but familiar feeling was overtaking me. I grew up in a home where it was dangerous to feel too much pleasure. My parents seemed to experience my pleasure in experiences and people outside of our home as a kind of disloyalty. It was as if I weren't sufficiently appreciative of all that they provided. It was a short step in my unconscious to feeling that the group resented my wonderful vacation. It must have taken me about 5 minutes to sort out all these feeling and attend to what was actually taking place in the group. I could now feel that the group was glad to see me.

My countertransference sorted out, three quarters of the way through the 80-minute group, I commented on this seating arrangement *that was unusual for this group*—since no one else had. Ordinarily, even with several absences, group members would routinely sit on either side of me. Mike, Roberta, and Alyssa had all noticed the seating pattern but had initially decided not to comment.

Mike and Alyssa then explained their seating decisions. Mike said that his fears of transparency kept him from sitting close to the leader. He was afraid that if he sat next to me, it would have been evident to the group how much he had missed me. Mike did not comment on the seating arrangement because he thought doing so would draw attention to the intensity of his dependency longings of which he was ashamed.

Alyssa mentioned that she needed a prescription filled while I was away and that the covering physician had taken two days to return her call. Alyssa, the group caretaker, felt conflicted making this disclosure. She was upset that she had to wait two days to get her anxiety medication but worried that in criticizing my covering person she would upset me. The inner conflict accounted for her sitting as far from me as possible. Alyssa did not mention the seating arrangement because she feared that the resulting discussion might annoy me and jeopardize our connection.

Roberta was too self-absorbed upon entering the group to pay attention to where she sat. She explained that her son, about to be a college junior, had a psychotic break while I was away. She was filled with shame and terror about what the future held for her family. She felt that the seating arrangement didn't seem important enough to comment on given her concerns about her son and her family. Time ran out before the other members had a chance to share their take on the seating arrangement.

In retrospect, if I hadn't been able to sort out my countertransference feelings, I might have mired the group in a discussion of negative feelings I imagined they harbored about my extended vacation. While there well might have been some feelings of abandonment, it was clear that the group was pleased to be together again and to have me back. The psychotherapeutic work the group accomplished—why they sat where they did and the feelings involved—was characteristic of a cohesive and working group.

Ted, a manager at a large computer company, consistently paid his group bill late. The group was not surprised to learn about his tardy payments because Ted had told the group that he often was charged a late fee on his credit card—even though he had the money to pay on time. As other group members handed me their checks at the beginning of the session, Ted would watch them paying me. What feelings, thoughts, or fantasies did he have as he took note of their paying on time? And wouldn't it seem like human nature that the other group members would wonder or even ask Ted that question? Since no one did, I asked Ted what it was like for him to watch other group members pay me. He wasn't surprised by the question. He said—and to his credit for being honest—that he thought of them as "brown-noses and goody-goodies." Sylvia asked him if that kind of condescension might have relevance at work where the people he supervised found him arrogant and difficult to work under. Ted's body posture and facial expression indicated that he took Sylvia's comment to heart.

Why did it take me so long to ask Ted about his experience as he watched other group members pay me on time when he never did? His behavior was there for everyone to observe—including me—but no one did, or if they did, they never commented on it. I think my not noticing had to do with a feeling of irritation that Ted evoked in me. His erratic manner of paying his bill resulted in bookkeeping errors that I would make, errors that resulted in my spending a lot of time rectifying these mistakes. A later exploration of Ted's inconsistent bill paying revealed a history of passive-aggressive behaviors dating back to his adolescence. Ted's father was a hard-driving businessman who spent little time with the family. Ted's attempts, through irritating behaviors, were no more successful in getting his father's attention than they were in obtaining the group's attention, including mine.

I've always been impressed with all the energy and thought that goes into the maintenance of omissions as well as the important information contained in them. Think of family members who, over a minor slight or miscommunication, don't talk with each other for years. It takes a lot of dedication to wake up every morning and remember not to talk to X—and yet there is usually so much to be talked about.

Group members begin to notice the important material revealed by tending to omissions. Over time, group members begin to internalize the leader's tendency to notice omissions—or to be interested in the feelings that interfered with noticing what was transpiring in the group. When a critical mass of group members has developed this ability, the group becomes an even more potent therapeutic agent.

"Get small and talk to the wall."

Many years ago, I was an examiner for the Board Examinations in Psychiatry. I evaluated the interviewing skills of a very intelligent, well-trained candidate whose task it was to interview a chronic schizophrenic patient. The interview was to last for an hour. This was obviously a very important moment in the candidate's professional life and he was eager to demonstrate his knowledge and ability. The patient, despite having been paid for his participation in the examination, appeared exhausted and no longer interested in cooperating. Four other candidates had interviewed the patient that day. It became clear to the candidate after five minutes that the patient had lost interest and had no intention of talking with him. The candidate looked away from the patient, assumed a beleaguered posture as he walked to and fro, and began thinking aloud in the room:

"I'm really upset and frustrated that I have prepared so long and hard for this exam and now Mr X will not even cooperate. I find myself becoming more concerned with my performance than with this man's welfare. Realizing this, I start to feel badly about myself because while this is an important day for me, Mr X appears to be a man who has struggled with major emotional difficulty for many years. I have gone into this field to help people like him and yet I now find myself resenting him, even wanting to hurt him. On the other hand, I don't want to infantilize him and exempt him from responsibility simply because he has mental problems. I do not know him well enough to know if he is unable or unwilling to cooperate."

The candidate continued speaking as honestly and openly as he could, revealing his inner struggle to remain in empathic contact with the patient and not to concern himself excessively with his performance on the exam. During this monologue the patient never looked at the candidate and seemed in his own world. When I indicated that time was up, the patient said "Good luck," a remark that lent itself to various interpretations: "Good luck, you'll need it" or "Good riddance" or "Best wishes." Judging from the patient's tone and demeanor and from the impression that the candidate's soliloquy made on me, I felt the patient meant to convey the following message, "I noticed how respectfully you treated me and I appreciate it. You deserve to pass your exam and I hope you do." (Of course, he passed!)

There are several noteworthy points in this example. Clearly the situation was very difficult for both the patient and the candidate. The patient was probably exhausted from the four previous interviews during which possibly upsetting material was discussed. The candidate was confronted with a situation that could negatively affect his future professionally. There seemed to be no opportunity to talk with the patient to improve the situation. Being able to put his many upsetting feelings into words probably contributed to the candidate's seeming emotional equanimity. Perhaps the very sound of his voice was soothing. Since the candidate's talking to the room in this particular context could be considered aberrant, it may have relaxed the patient by, so to speak, leveling the playing field. In spite of his conflicted feelings toward the patient, the candidate had managed both not to shame and to show respect for the patient, seeming to proceed on the assumption that the apparently unreachable patient was actually a sentient human being. The patient's parting comment highlighted the paradoxical nature of the situation: by not talking directly to the patient, the candidate had made a meaningful connection with him, a connection that most likely would not have occurred if he had persisted in trying to get the patient to talk. The soliloquy also helped the candidate avoid a common therapist mistake, namely, medicating one's feeling of powerlessness by trying to control another person.

I became intrigued with the therapeutic technique "get small and talk to the wall" as I realized that it could be helpful when therapy has reached an impasse. An extremely painful feeling with which the patient struggles is often, though not always, the cause of the impasse. The unbearable feeling inevitably and necessarily involves the therapist and distorts the therapy in a variety of ways. Consider the following situations. Massive and unresolved disappointment in a parent resurfaces in the patient's disappointment in the therapist, a disappointment profound enough to threaten the therapy with an abrupt unilateral termination. Unbearable loneliness, enough to be life-threatening, presents as paranoia. The paranoia is a desperate attempt to medicate the loneliness with the belief that I'm not alone, that I'm constantly watched albeit by a hostile world. The therapist becomes caught in a projected beam of suspicion from the patient from which there appears to be no escape. A person immobilized by ambivalence seeks therapy. Gradually the patient's wish to be in therapy is replaced by the patient's belief that she is continuing in therapy only at her therapist's insistence. The patient feels intense resentment.

All of these scenarios place the therapist in a very difficult position. How is the therapist to be a helpful presence when the patient experiences the therapist as no longer competent, safe, or respectful? The therapist's self-image as a helper and the patient's sense of the therapist as a disappointment, a threatening presence, or a controlling other, create a potentially unworkable situation. In the patient's eyes the therapist takes on a large, dominant, and dangerous presence. The therapist must come up with a different and novel way to proceed. The therapist needs to get out of the patient's line of vision or else continue to be an object of the patient's negative projections. One part of the attempted solution is for the therapist to talk to the room while not looking at the patient. The other part of the attempted solution is for the therapist to take on a smaller presence. The therapist accomplishes this stance through tone of voice (beleaguered), body posture (slumped), and a mock retreat into soliloquy.

The aversion of gaze is another component of the therapist's getting "smaller." Dominance can be achieved through eye contact, a behavior in which the therapist elects not to engage. By eschewing eye contact, the patient is empowered to take up more space. Since eye contact also secures the attention of the other, projection often follows attention. By withdrawing eye contact, the therapist also seeks to avoid being the object of the patient's projections because people tend to believe their projections. It will only make matters worse if the patient is allowed to locate in the therapist the negative feelings he/she is presently overwhelmed with. Thus, the therapist, while talking to the room, looks out the window or at the floor or the wall. The therapist's actual positioning may be such that the patient sees the top of the therapist's head or profile. Highly touted eye contact is not always therapeutic.

Therapists' soliloquies consist of countertransference use for therapeutic purposes.[2] The topics spoken about vitally concern their patients. Therapists deliver their soliloquies as empathically or thoughtfully as possible, according to their overall estimation of the therapeutic requirements of the moment. In their soliloquies therapists may reframe emotional difficulties that their patient has induced in them as attempts at communication. For example, 1 therapist may suggest that the patient has induced in her the same feeling the patient is presently overwhelmed with in the hope that she will develop greater empathy for the patient. Another therapist, responding to the same emotional reactions, may decide that the patient would benefit from hearing about his actual inner experience in relation to the patient. And yet a 3rd therapist might soliloquize over her frustration while pursuing directly a perpetually elusive patient.

Winnicott proposed that psychotherapy takes place in the overlap of 2 areas of playing, that of the patient and that of therapist.[3] When such play is no longer possible, when it breaks down, the therapist tries to bring the patient from a state of not being able to play into a state of being able to play.

Abrupt unilateral termination in therapy is a good example of where a mutual state of play in therapy has broken down. Both parties are in emotional pain. The patient has invested time, money, energy, and hope in a therapy that has disappointed. Most likely the patient is filled with painful feelings that, for one reason or another, were not addressed and resolved. The therapist is faced with sudden abandonment, loss of income, and a possible threat to feelings of competence, especially if the therapy seemed to be going well. The therapist may feel any number of the following: caught off guard, angry, unfairly treated, abandoned, relieved, abused, unloved, and, frequently, de-skilled.

The therapist may wish to analyze the patient's resistance but doing so may prove difficult because of the many negative feelings that have been stirred up in the therapist. Appealing to the therapeutic alliance is also not an option because the patient has already violated a fundamental rule of therapy: to talk about important decisions before acting on them. Talking about the patient's wish to leave at this point would amount to pseudo-therapy. What needs to be talked about before addressing any other topics is why the patient decided to make the decision to leave without first talking to his therapist. The therapist realizes that, unfortunately, such an option is not viable; the patient is mainly intent on ending the therapy. Talking to the room may be the only possibility left to the therapist at this point. Here is an example.

Sid felt that I disapproved of an affair he had while dating a serious girlfriend— which wasn't true. He announced without any warning that this would be his last session. He had just received an important promotion at work that far surpassed his hated father's middle management position. Assuming an oppressed posture, I began thinking aloud in the room without looking at him. "Let's see, I recall that Sid was furious at his father for selling his mother's car without first discussing with her his intention to do so . . . so many things have not turned out well for Sid: his parents' stormy divorce during his adolescence, never having a relationship with his younger brother, his recent break-up with his girlfriend. I guess it's not surprising that his therapy should prove to be a disappointment as well."

Silence. I continued, "I can't blame Sid for wanting to leave therapy because at this rate he is likely to have a better life than his father." From the other side of the room he said, "My life is already better than my father's." I agreed with him, saying, "It's true, one thing that Sid has that his father doesn't is an awareness of his own sadness." With one minute left in the session, Sid asked me what I thought. I told him that I thought we were out of time and that I would see him next week. He said that there wasn't going to be any next time. I did not accept his offer of a handshake as he left.

I wrote Sid a brief note stating that I thought he needed to come back and talk about his sudden decision to leave. He returned for 3 sessions and we talked about his anger, expressed in the repeated pattern of finding other people inadequate, unfair, or judgmental. He decided to see someone else but said he was glad that I didn't let him terminate unilaterally. He acknowledged that he was leaving me with a greater appreciation of the role he plays in not letting other people's interest in and responsiveness to him ever be sufficient. A year later I received a note from him in which he commented on the following paradox: it was only when I decided not to speak to him directly that he was first able to hear what I had been trying to say directly to him for weeks.

Notes

1 Luft, J. (1966). *An Introduction to Group Dynamics*. Palo Alto, CA: National Press.
2 Gans, J. S. (1994). Indirect communication as a therapeutic technique: A novel use of counter transference. *Amer J Psychother*, 48: 120–140.
3 Winnicott, D. W. (1960). *Maturational Process and the Facilitating Environment*. New York: International University Press, Inc.

Chapter 15

Responding therapeutically to patients' questions

To a patient who frequently requests that I do something: "How would you feel if I did what you asked and how would you feel if I declined to do what you asked?"

Psychotherapy patients sometimes ask their therapists to undertake an action on their behalf. "Would you testify at my disability hearing?" "Would you attend my wedding?" "Would you meet for a double session?" "Would you read my term paper?"

Beginning therapists find such requests unsettling for several reasons. They are concerned that if they decline to "do something," their patients will be offended, dislike them or feel disliked by them, or even terminate therapy. More familiar with the institution of friendship than the workings of therapy, neophyte therapists feel awkward in declining to do for a patient what they would naturally do for a friend.

A basic rule of therapy assists therapists with this dilemma: Requests for action are to be explored before any decision regarding action is made. Not unlike a railroad crossing, "Stop, Look, and Listen" are useful guides. The three major effects of this rule are monumental. First, it helps guard against beginning therapists' tendency to focus exclusively on external reality and to act or to explain rather than to explore. Second, the emphasis on exploration serves to shift the locus of patients' and therapists' attention from external reality to their respective internal worlds. Third, it implants the notion that there are "out-of-awareness" processes at work that need to be explored.

George asked his fledgling female therapist to read his lengthy term paper, which she agreed to do on her own time. Shortly thereafter, she felt upset with herself for having agreed, but didn't know exactly why. Supervision brought several of her concerns to consciousness. She realized that she felt coerced into agreeing to read the term paper by her fear that if she didn't, George, to whom she felt attracted, would leave the therapy. Having agreed to read the paper, what would she do if she thought the paper was poorly done? Could she, would she, actually tell him? And if she did, would he feel criticized and/or rejected? She also realized that she resented not getting paid for spending her private time gratis and

DOI: 10.4324/9781003174608-19

yet, what could she do? After all *she* had agreed. Or was it permissible for her to broach the possibility of getting paid for her time? And finally, had she unwittingly opened the door to further requests for special attention?

Supervision helped this therapist appreciate that her expertise resided in her ability to explore thoughts, feelings, and fantasies—both her patient's and, silently, her own. She returned to the therapy excited and now equipped with questions that helped her explore her patient's internal world and the therapist–patient relationship: "What would it be like for you if I liked your paper, and what would it be like for you if I didn't?" "How did you fear I would react?" "How did you hope I would react?" "What was it like for you to ask me to read your paper?" "Even though I didn't ask, did you think I should be compensated for the time I spent reading it?" And, "Could it be that you have other requests that you have not yet shared with me?" Also, as a result of talking in supervision about her attraction to her patient, she no longer felt uncomfortable. Her feelings of attraction had lost their sense of urgency and became just another topic to be explored and understood.

Exploration produced changes in the therapy hour over time. George seemed less preoccupied with news of the week or other people's psychology. He was more conscious of his longings and began to realize that real therapy consisted of exploring those wishes rather than expecting his therapist to fulfill them. His capacity for introspection increased. The therapist noticed that she was no longer uptight about the consequences of whether or not she liked her patient's paper, or whether or not she would be paid. She enjoyed her attraction to George rather than being unsettled by it. She gained a clearer appreciation of what patients value the most in therapy: being understood rather than catered to, attaining self-knowledge through heightened introspection, and the therapist's compassionate neutrality and firm, non-judgmental maintenance of boundaries.

Therapy proceeds by working through layers of material, even for the same issue. George indirectly indicated by making yet another request of his therapist that his wish for special attention still required further psychotherapeutic work. He asked her twice to write a letter excusing him from work for psychological reasons, one time for a bout of depression that in fact was not that debilitating. His therapist encouraged him to explore his thoughts, feelings, and fantasies connected to his request. This suggestion led George to recall a turbulent period in his early teens precipitated by his mother's affair that had disrupted family life. Dark clouds suddenly spoiled what had felt like a carefree upbringing. Although the marriage survived, he blamed his mother for ruining his adolescence. He wanted restitution: "Mother, I expect you to make up to me the period of my life that you ruined." Despite making yet another request, George knew by now that his therapist would encourage him to explore the feelings driving the request; he knew, and at some level was reassured by knowing, that she would not act on his request.

Another example shows how gratifying a patient's atypical request can lead to poor results. After his female therapist agreed to extend Alex's session for 5 minutes, he besieged her (nicely) with additional requests. Could she change the time of his appointment (on several occasions); accept delayed payment for therapy sessions; write a letter explaining why he should be exempted from jury duty, etc.? While indulging these requests, his therapist found herself annoyed by Alex's feeling of entitlement. Who does he think he is, some privileged character? Most likely, Alex, in making these requests was just being himself, oblivious to the likelihood that this pattern of requests had significance in his life. As Scott Rutan has so often said, patients do not present with problems, rather they present with solutions.[1] This was obviously a solution Alex had used for years. The therapist's gratification of Alex's requests reinforced his ego-syntonic behavior. She unwittingly made it less likely that Alex would be invested in becoming self-conscious or curious about the behavior since, after all, both people in the office had seen nothing remarkable about it over an extended period of time. The therapist's growing sense of impatience or annoyance at these multiple requests, and her growing dissatisfaction with herself for indulging them, made it more difficult for her to maintain a posture of curiosity as opposed to judgment. When his therapist finally was able to ask him if he had ever been curious about the number of special requests he had made of her, he replied with some justification, "Not really, you've given me no reason to think the requests have been out of the ordinary or have bothered you." The therapist had squandered therapeutic leverage she would have had if from the beginning she had fostered in her patient a sense of curiosity about this emerging pattern rather than immediately acting on his requests.

The secure and trusting relationship I had with this supervisee allowed us to consider the concept of projective identification. We speculated on—but resisted a deeper exploration more appropriate for therapy—what it was about *her* that allowed the indulgence of her male patient's sense of entitlement.

"How did you think about the question your patient just asked you?" (spoken to my supervisee)

This query is more complicated than it seems because there are so many aspects of a patient's question to consider. It has been my experience that neophyte therapists especially benefit from this supervisory question.

First, does the question feel like a question? Let's assume that at the start of the therapy the therapist explained that questions will be answered when, in the therapist's professional opinion, it is in the patient's best interest to do so. A real question can be as easily answered as not. When it feels like the question must be answered, what is being asked is not a question but a demand. A demand involves coercion. The content of the demand is less significant than the coercion, which requires exploration. Here are some examples: "You don't believe me, do you?" "Don't you agree that my wife was at fault?" "The other people in the group get a lot more attention than I do—right?" "You agree that I'm ready to terminate, don't you?" "You have doubts that I was sexually molested, right? Well, you don't deny it, do you?"

The coercion embedded in these examples suggests that they are not real questions. The person asking the question expects—often demands—instant agreement. "If you are not entirely with me, then you are against me" is often the meta-communication. No time is allowed for the gathering of more information. Demanding agreement is much different from being a willing collaborator in pursuing the truth—with a small *t*. The demand for agreement constitutes an unwitting self-disclosure: the demander conducts business through power and coercion rather than collaboration and exploration.

If the patient is asking a real question, the therapist must decide if, when, and how to answer. Answering a question immediately usually provides gratification that lessens the patient's motivation to do the work of self-examination. But that is not always the case. Some patients need immediate answers that facilitate the introspection that therapy requires. For example, some patients feel shamed if their question is responded to with a question. These patients receive direct answers as a sign of respect and experience their therapists as optimally responsive. This responsiveness provides the impetus these patients need to do the work of psychotherapy.

There is a situation where questions that are not real questions are not coercive. Some patients who call on the phone for a first appointment have question after question for the prospective therapist: "Where is your office?" "Do you have another office that is closer to where I work?" "How long have you been in practice?" "What is your theoretical orientation?" "Where were you trained?" "How long does it take to get to your office during peak traffic from downtown?" "Do you see patients in the evening or on weekends?" The therapist who is still on the phone fielding these questions will most likely not get to see this patient in therapy. In most cases, this seemingly endless stream of questions represents massive ambivalence toward therapy by a patient who often cancels the first appointment.

Novice and veteran patients have different expectations and responses to having their questions answered. Patients beginning dynamic therapy and unaccustomed to its culture may initially expect their questions to be answered, especially if their therapist has not explained at the start of therapy how he/she conducts the sessions. They experience their questions not being answered as a sign of rudeness and disrespect. Veteran patients may well expect that the content of the question and why it was asked will be explored before the therapist decides whether to answer it. Veteran patients may be surprised by an immediate answer and, for the most part, feel deprived of the usual opportunity for self-reflection.

One of the most challenging questions for a therapist to answer honestly without shaming the patient or losing credibility is "What do you think of me?" Notice all the possibilities the therapist might consider before answering or not. Why is the patient asking this question at this particular time? The patient might have just revealed something shameful, has sensed disapproval from the therapist, and wants to check out his reality testing. The patient may be overly self-critical and has projected this tendency onto the therapist. The patient may need reassurance that he is not disliked, a feeling he needs in so many other situations in his life.

Perhaps his therapist has just returned from a long vacation that the patient has experienced as abandonment. The patient wonders if it was something about him that kept his therapist away for so long. Or is the question a distraction from something that would be more difficult for the patient to talk about: *what he thinks of his therapist*? Attention to the patient's tone—pleading, challenging, fearful, earnest, anxious, or sad—helps the therapist decide which of these possibilities to address.

Consider the challenging question, "What effect do I have on you?" which a difficult male patient asks his female therapist. She would do well to consider a number of pitfalls before responding to this question. Will I dispense criticism rather than compassionately neutral feedback? Will my answer betray my preference for a compliant patient rather than a patient who causes discomfort? Is the question a set-up, a "when did you stop beating your wife" type of question, for which there is no answer that will satisfy the patient? What if there is an erotic current in the therapy that the therapist has not sufficiently metabolized?

Let us consider a situation in which an experienced therapist's response to a real question could be therapeutic. A patient with a history replete with examples of irresponsibility, and who has been in therapy for 3 years, suddenly asks her therapist, "You don't trust me, do you?" The therapist might be afraid that a truthful answer would jeopardize the alliance. An untruthful answer, however, might be just as damaging because at some level the patient knows she is irresponsible. The challenge is to be truthful without being shaming or judgmental. A possible reply is, "Of course I don't trust you—sometimes. I sense that my distrust of you results from your distrust of yourself. Part of our work together is to learn more about what your self-distrust is all about."

Several aspects of this response can strengthen the therapeutic alliance. The therapist is demonstrating thoughtfulness: I do think about what transpires in here. I'm not taking your unreliability personally. I am trying to be honest without being unnecessarily hurtful. You probably would wonder about me if I said I trust you, since, after all, your distrust of yourself is a major problem that brought you into therapy. We are working on this together, and, you should know, there are times when I do trust you (you are not irredeemably undependable).

A third example: Bill rarely missed a group meeting, arrived at meetings on time, paid his bill promptly, and asked other people useful questions. However, he rarely took risks or self-disclosed personal material, despite the group's interest in him. He spoke in a monotone that caused other members to tune him out. One day, Bill, uncharacteristically, looked directly at me and asked, "What do you think of me?" In a reply that I appropriated from a respected colleague, I said, "I guess I think of you as an annuity." Laughter erupted and Bill looked at first confused and then hurt. He asked what I meant and I asked the other group members what they made of my comment. I did so partly to take the spotlight off Bill. Various group members commented on how they sometimes experienced Bill as more of a fixture in the room than a person interested in working on himself, despite his interest in others. Others objected to my comment that they experienced as demeaning.

Still others said they were reassured by my honesty. They thought that I could never have made such a comment if I was comfortable exploiting Bill, taking his money and not caring if he did any emotional work. The content of subsequent sessions indicated that my comment had served as a kind of shock treatment. Bill began talking about his dissatisfaction with his dead-end job and the fact that he had still not unpacked some of the boxes in his apartment that he had moved into 2 years ago. In retrospect, I think Bill was able to take my comment to heart partly because of the playful manner in which it was delivered. I also think Bill got my message, "I don't want to exploit you. I prefer that you do the work of therapy. As you do the work of therapy, I will feel better about getting paid."

In friendship, for the most part, questions are taken and responded to at face value. In therapy, questions have a variety of motives. They are generated by a wide range of feelings and arise at various stages of therapy. In responding, the therapist must be sensitive to language and respond in ways that are honest, believable, and in the service of the patient's needs and growth. The supervisory question "How did you think about the question your patient just asked you?" provides the supervisee an opportunity to think more deeply about the many therapeutic challenges such questions pose.

Note

1   Rutan, S. (2005). Personal communication.

Chapter 16

Securing the patient's attention

"You are a serial killer."

It's amazing the things a therapist has to say sometimes to get a patient's attention. It seems counterintuitive that telling a patient "You are a serial killer" could be potentially therapeutic. Of course, such a statement is made with sensitivity to timing, vulnerability, and receptivity combined with the caring explanation "You are accomplished in killing off continuity and, more tragically, parts of yourself."

Some patients start every session as if no sessions had ever preceded it. *They kill off continuity*. They short-circuit the very therapy they have sought out. I see 32 patient hours/week and remembered something Ed told me from the last session. I brought up the incident in the next session and Ed didn't remember having mentioned it. Not surprisingly, Ed came upon his ability to "annihilate" honestly. Ed's father, a disbarred lawyer, told him repeatedly during his adolescence that he would never amount to much. Ever the "devoted" son, Ed fulfilled his father's prediction. As a salesman for a computer company, he forfeited thousands of dollars by failing to submit his travel expenses for reimbursement in a timely way. He antagonized his boss and was never promoted. He was unfaithful in his childless marriage, which resulted in divorce. A bitterness that permeated many sectors of his life alienated his few remaining friends. Rebelling against dietary restrictions imposed by his childhood diabetes, he became obese and at age 49 suffered a mild stroke during his third year in therapy. Telling Ed that he was a "serial killer" and using a word like annihilate to characterize his killing off friendships provided a kind of non-electric shock treatment that helped him take a hard look at his relentless negativity and self-destructive behaviors.

Beatrice entered therapy for the treatment of anxiety and announced matter-of-factly that when her older sister, Ellen, who had cancer, died, she was going to kill herself. Her therapist, who was my supervisee, became preoccupied with this disturbing threat. We spent many months in supervision trying to gain a better understanding of the patient as well as the supervisee's countertransference. What slowly came into focus was that for all intents and purposes Beatrice was already dead. She had no friends and no family except for Ellen. She had no sense of a future and was guilt ridden about her past. In the present she existed rather than

DOI: 10.4324/9781003174608-20

lived. She had no imagination or, if she had one, she refused to use it. She hated her body and had no sexual feelings for years. Nothing gave her pleasure. She reported that she never had dreams. She was sure that her death would have no impact on her therapist.

Beatrice's self-destructiveness had a profound effect on her therapist who became unnerved by an image his patient had evoked in him. He had a fleeting, ego-dystonic image of slicing his wrists with a knife. That image alerted him to how much of Beatrice's rage he was holding and containing. The therapist was then able to suggest to Beatrice that if she could feel this rage and put some of it into words, hopefully she wouldn't have to direct so much of it at herself. The therapist said, "You keep telling me about your plans to kill yourself in the future. I'm concerned about how much of yourself you are killing off right now."

What kinds of early life experiences give rise to this kind of "serial killing?" I envision a child of two sitting on her depressed mother's lap before getting down to go off and play. Pleasurable exploration immediately gives way to inner conflict and constraint. Even at this early stage of development, the child knows it is not "nice" to leave her depressed mother who, the child feels, will dislike her for leaving. Knowing that she cannot survive without her mother's love and afraid she is jeopardizing it by abandoning her, she is too anxious and fearful to be self-possessed and to feel curious. To escape the designation of "bad child,"—her punishment for abandoning her mother—she returns to her mother feigning contentment at the expense of spontaneity and authenticity. She is riddled with guilt and conflict. She has sacrificed herself on the altar of her mother's fragility. Her raison d'être becomes the maintenance of her mother's intactness if not her survival. Pleasurable exploration immediately gives way to guilt and self-constraint. She is to take care of others at the expense of herself. She is not to experience pleasure, either in her body or her relationships. Some satisfaction is permitted at work as long as she puts other people's needs before her own.

Patients I have treated who have this profile report the following childhood feelings. They felt invisible, overlooked, unprotected, and least favored. They were mistreated and eclipsed by siblings. Parents provided little to no safety. They felt an inordinate need to be very, very good. These children "trained" others to exploit them, all the while seething with resentment over not being acknowledged and appreciated. They kept the bitterness suppressed with compulsive good deeds. As adults, they are suffused with guilt about all their resentments. Their suppressed and projected anger makes other people feel too dangerous to be close to. Their wish for connections with others atrophied. If they did call others, their phone hardly ever rung in return. They were unable to cry at funerals; they never felt loved enough by people to miss them. As time went on, their bitterness and rage weakened many of their strengths and connections with others. They ended up doing to themselves as adults what was done to them as children. They became mostly benumbed by a feeling of aloneness that otherwise would have been too painful to bear. They became the walking dead, known to the world as nice people, if in fact they were nice. At the same time, they are usually extremely honest, trustworthy, intelligent, and generous, albeit burdened with ambivalence.

While long-term therapy with these folks can bring them back to life, it is a very, very slow process. Two juxtaposed memories illustrate my work over the years with Anita, who had one younger sister. In one image, at age 15, she is coming down in a hospital elevator with her father who was recovering from a below-the-knee amputation. His physical therapist, who had worked with him for over 3 months, was in the elevator. Her father introduced her to the physical therapist, who said, "I never knew you had another daughter." In the other image, which occurred a few decades later, Anita entered the session with a sense of triumph and self-satisfaction. She had overcome a lifelong inhibition. As a girl and young woman, anytime she wanted to buy something for herself her mother would say critically, "Why do you need that?" In the past, she would always deny herself. With a wide smile and excitement I had never before witnessed, she showed me a pair of diamond stud earrings that she had purchased for herself. That image of Anita is forever etched in my mind. The therapy had helped her develop a sense of self-worth. She started to feel that she deserved some good things in life. She could now direct energy that had formerly gone into self-annihilation into behaviors that gave her some pleasure. She was no longer a "serial killer."

"You don't treat your help very well."

Imagine a successful career at midlife despite the stresses of young children and aging, infirm parents. You accept a new patient, Harold, regardless of the fact that your demanding psychotherapy practice is more than full. Harold turns out to be a pious hypocrite who attends Mass every morning and does his thing as a predatory slum landlord for the rest of the day. An expert at offering unsolicited advice, he seems refractory to self-examination. Because of your excellent reputation and the convenience of your office's location, he accepts your missed session and cancellation policy that holds the patient financially responsible—even though he feels the policy is unfair. Although he endured a childhood of physical abuse and neglect, you find it very hard to like Harold. Feeling stifled by the weekly therapy schedule, he begins missing sessions, promising to pay for them, always having a self-justifying excuse why he hasn't. He begins to demean your therapeutic approach. The pattern goes on for two months. Frustrated, aware of the tenuous therapeutic alliance, depleted of empathy for Harold, you say to him, "You don't treat your help very well." In a telephone call two days later, he informs you that he is stopping therapy. Somewhat relieved, you look forward to using the statement "You don't treat your help very well" to better advantage in the future with a more workable patient who also resents all the power he feels you unfairly exert.

A power differential exists in psychodynamic psychotherapy: the therapist possesses significantly more of it than the patient does. The therapist charges the patient a fee for the meetings and sets a missed session and cancellation policy; indicates the purpose of the meetings; chooses the location (her office), the frequency of the sessions, and, often, the time when she and the patient will meet.

Compared to patient self-disclosures, the therapist reveals comparatively little about herself. In most instances, the therapist assumes more importance in the patient's life than the patient does in the therapist's life—although the therapist's caring for the patient is substantial. Therapists possess something of great value— love that, at some level of consciousness, patients long for and know they have to pay for. And finally, the therapist, hopefully, understands more about the patient than the patient understands about himself—especially in the beginning phases of the therapy. Contrast these inequalities with friendship where the power held by each party is usually more or less equal.

Once transference takes hold, it seems to the patient that the therapist accrues even more power. Originally the patient sought out treatment for a particular problem. As time passes the patient's decision to seek therapy often morphs into the patient's feeling that the therapist prefers his continued participation in the process. Remaining in therapy can even come to feel like the therapist's demand, rather than the patient's decision. Further increasing the therapist's apparent degree of power is a subtle but powerful dynamic that begins to dominate the therapy: the patient, who initially came for relief of suffering and a better under- standing of his problems, now finds that his wish to be loved or at least cared for and respected by his therapist takes on an overwhelming importance.

Over time a powerful fiction takes hold: the therapist possesses all the power. The fact that some therapists act as if, or believe, this is true should not obscure another reality: the patient also has considerable power in the therapy. Without patients, therapists would have no practice. Without patients who are motivated to work on their problems, or motivated to work on their resistance to working on their problems, therapists may have a body in the office but not (yet) an actual psychotherapy patient. Therapists' self-esteem depends to a certain degree on patients who value therapy provided by caring, competent, and dependable clini- cians. This fact has been brought into focus during the pandemic where therapists and patients share basic existential issues. Because of this shifting of the playing field, and because other concerns assume greater importance in patients' lives— like staying alive—therapists, while still important to their patients, become less important and, consequently have less power. To the extent that therapists experi- ence the decrease in high regard in which their patients formerly held them, thera- pists may suffer a loss of a sense of power. (There is an exception to this pattern. My supervisees report that patients who live alone often feel an increased need for their therapists during the pandemic, seem to value them more, and sometimes wish to meet more frequently. As a result, these therapists feel both more highly valued and—finding it hard to refuse their patients' requests for more frequent visits—more exhausted.)

It is in the financial realm that patients wield their greatest power. Patients pay our salary and decide, in leaving us, when they will no longer pay us. It never occurs to some patients who pay their bill sporadically, consistently late, or, in a few cases, never, that their therapists actually depend on their money. Telling them, when the timing seems right, "You don't treat your help very well," has a way of alerting them to power that they actually possess. Referring to herself as "your help," a status usually associated with a person with less power, the therapist both catches the patient off guard and, by contrast, elevates the patient's standing vis-à-vis the therapist: "You're my boss, you hire me, and I work for you." Bosses don't conjure up visions of powerless victims.

Some patients, for whom it is important not to register the business part of the relationship, experience therapists as acting solely out of benevolence. I became more aware of this dynamic at a cocktail party when I overheard someone say that his cardiologist "*gave* me an electrocardiogram." A bystander piped up and said, "No, she *sold* you an electrocardiogram." The obliviousness with which these patients—as is their prerogative as patients—treat our imagined finances can have a surprisingly powerful effect, especially on therapists not tuned into the transferential aspects of this behavior or to those therapists experiencing financial difficulties.

Paying our salary and terminating our employment are only part of the power that patients possess. The feelings that attend the financial transaction can be a force to be reckoned with. Many feelings get attached to money that have nothing to do with money per se. In withholding or delaying payment, the patient may be indirectly or directly communicating a variety of feelings to the therapist, either consciously or, often, unconsciously. Here are a few of the messages they might be conveying:

- "You won't love me if I don't pay you, will you? See, your caring is fake."
- "You take my money but give me nothing. See how you like it when I withhold your fee."
- "You need to make up to me all that I have been deprived of and until you do, I'm not paying."
- "This therapy depletes me; I have nothing left to give you."
- "I want to hurt you (back) financially."
- "You call this therapy (said derisively) and yet I have to pay for it."

When therapists are tuned into the transferential nature of these communications and interpret them empathically, the therapy is usually advanced and therapists, not having taken these messages personally, are not dislodged from their usual therapeutic posture. On the other hand, therapists' defenses and protective role can be overwhelmed when such indictments are relentless, highly personalized, spitefully conveyed, and refractory to interpretation. Therapists tend to be ashamed of the many thoughts, feelings, and fantasies that such assaults evoke. As a result, many of their feelings do not get discussed or processed.

An exception to such avoidance has occurred in my psychotherapy consultation group where this subject has come to be a lively topic of conversation. The therapists seem relieved to have a safe venue in which to discuss their countertransference. Interestingly, many of their unfriendly, hostile, and retaliatory thoughts and feelings emerged during a discussion of contemplating raising their fee for certain patients. Invariably these are patients who are having a powerful and destabilizing effect on them. Here are a few examples: "I notice when I consider raising my fee, it's always Ethel's fee I think of raising first. I really don't like her." "I should get $600/hour, not $200/hour for treating Sam. He's such a demanding, very difficult patient." "It doesn't bother me when some people haven't paid me, but with Mary, I want my money now. I really do, I guess what I want is my pound of flesh."

Successful therapies are ones where, at their conclusion, a more equitable distribution of power is achieved. Paying attention to the powerful emotional currents that attend financial transactions in therapy provides an opportunity to alert patients to the power that they do possess. The statement, "You don't treat your help well," where appropriate and with sensitive timing, can assist patients in claiming a sense of agency.

Chapter 17

Dealing with the group's resistance

"I'm concerned about *poor* Gloria. How outrageous will she have to act before someone recognizes her behavior and is willing to talk with her about it?"

It is remarkable the kinds of behavior some families are willing to tolerate, encourage, or ignore. A 16-year-old boy has an affair with his 38-year-old female social studies teacher and emerges from the caper a local hero in his male peer group. His parents react by saying, "Oh, boys will be boys, Henry is a good kid." Another family tolerates with impunity their mother's sense of entitlement. She drives through tollbooths without paying, saying that she can't be bothered. In an even more egregious example, a family notes that one of its elder members eats food on only one-half of his plate. Another family member turns the plate 180 degrees so he can finish his meal. One day they find him urinating in the kitchen sink, apparently mistaking it for a toilet. It is only after he carves "Fuck you" on the treasured family piano that they decide to bring him to the family doctor. (And yes, this really did happen!)

Some people, as they emerge from their families of origin and enter the adult world, proceed as if the world functions in accord with the atypical norms in their families. This mistaken presumption often leads to painful interpersonal and social difficulties.

One of the premises of psychodynamic group psychotherapy is that problematic behaviors that a person exhibits in the world will, if things go well, resurface in his/her group therapy relationships where they can be processed with kindness, compassion, and understanding. For example, a person prone to self-absorption will find it difficult to stay focused on another group member's story and will instead try to find a way to bring the group's attention to him. At some point, members of the group will be annoyed by this behavior—a form of stealing—and bring it to the person's attention. Group annoyance usually gives way to concern and compassion as the group learns more about the person and realizes that either he is unaware of this behavior or, if he is aware of it, that he cannot control it. The group begins to take this behavior less personally for two reasons. First, it gradually becomes clear that such behavior is problematic in other sectors of the

DOI: 10.4324/9781003174608-21

patient's life. Second, it has caused enough angst for this person to seek or be referred to group therapy.

In the following example, I will discuss how the statement in the chapter heading attempts to bring about heightened self and group awareness.

Gloria is a member of a "Process Group Experience" Institute at a national group psychotherapy conference, a 2-day, 13-hour encounter where the group studies its own process. Members of the group are all mental health practitioners with similar amounts of clinical experience. Being veterans of this type of group, they understand (only too well) that they are expected to arrive on time and stay for the entire experience. Gloria comes late to the morning and afternoon sessions of the first day. Her wristwatch beeps every hour on the hour, visibly annoying other group members, although no one comments on the distraction. An hour before the end of the afternoon session on the first day, Gloria announces that she has to leave early to pick up her daughter from day care, an egregious violation of the group contract that she has agreed to. She is also late to the morning session of the second day. An hour into this session, when no one has yet commented on Gloria's behavior, I say, "I'm concerned about *poor* Gloria. How outrageous will she have to be before someone recognizes her behavior and is willing to talk with her about it?"

The group now focuses on Gloria in an attempt to learn what her provocative behavior is all about. She provides some personal history. Since her stormy adolescence, she has had little contact with her Holocaust-survivor parents. When she was 15, her father gave her a book about the Holocaust to read. A week later he said to her, "So?" She answered, "So what!" at which point her father slapped her across the face. A group member says to Gloria, "Am I to understand from your story that the only way we can have a relationship with you is to react angrily to your behavior? Hopefully we can find a better way to relate to you." Gloria becomes noticeably sad after this comment and her disruptive behaviors markedly diminish.

My intervention—"I'm concerned about *poor* Gloria. How outrageous will she have to be before someone recognizes her behavior and is willing to talk with her about it?"—fosters group work in the following ways by:

1   focusing the spotlight not on Gloria's behavior but on the group's resistance to dealing with her;
2   empathizing ("poor Gloria") with the extent to which she has to go to get the group's attention;
3   implying that there seems to be a "courage deficiency" in the other group members, thereby inviting them to work harder;
4   assuring the group, by implication, that they have a leader who will be there for them if and when they are overlooked by the group;
5   reassuring Gloria that, despite the disruptions she has caused, she continues to have the leader's concern;
6   transforming the group into a "family" that, rather than punishing Gloria, seeks to understand what it was like to grow up in a home with Holocaust survivor parents.

You might be wondering why group members did not comment on Gloria's behavior. My remark indirectly invited group members to share their process in deciding to remain silent and not deal with Gloria's provocations. Group members had a range of different responses. Melanie said she knew and liked Gloria from time spent with her in previous Institutes and didn't want to shame her by calling out her behavior. George said that he was so irritated by Gloria that he was worried that whatever he said would be too judgmental. Alex said that this Institute was one of the most contentious he had ever been in and he didn't want to make things worse by focusing on Gloria. He felt that the group needed to build cohesion by sharing similar experiences. Elizabeth said that she trusted the leader to intervene when the time seemed right. Virginia said she had a history of stirring up trouble in Institutes and that she was relieved that Gloria had assumed that role. Steven commented on the educational function of Institutes and said he wanted to see how a senior group therapist would handle Gloria's provocative behavior. John said that he shared Melanie's wish not to shame Gloria and appreciated the leader's taking the spotlight off her and focusing on the members of the group.

"It is at times like this that I am so grateful for our (group) contract."

In evaluating and preparing a patient for participation in a therapy group, the group leader discusses and enlarges on the terms in the group contract, which include one's attendance, payment, confidentiality, out of group contact, and termination. Even though prospective group patients rarely say they find the terms troubling, experience has shown that after several months some members of the group will violate items in the contract. Why does this happen?

Group members tend to experience the group contract as a set of rules to which strict obedience is expected, even though such is not the case. The leader does not expect or require obedience to the contract. The leader expects that if and when uncomfortable feelings do *not* get talked about and processed, patients will violate the group contract. The prospective group members' acceptance of the group contract (in the pre-group evaluation) gives the leader leverage to expect the group member to take responsibility for any violation. Taking responsibility means that the offending group member will speak as openly and honestly as possible about the uncomfortable, unexpressed thoughts and feelings that gave rise to the violation. The discussion of the previously avoided feelings is what ultimately contributes to a sense of trust and safety in the group. Leaders who do not promote such discussions find that their groups are marked by unilateral terminations and/or spotty attendance.

The rule about termination is especially noteworthy. In joining the group, a member agrees "to let the group participate in the decision to terminate when I think the time has come to terminate, and to leave enough time to say good-bye once the decision to terminate has been made." During the 48 years that I have led weekly, out-patient, open-ended, psychodynamically oriented groups in my private practice, fewer than ten patients have terminated in the fashion that the contract prescribes.

More frequently members announce their decision to terminate and then indicate that they are open to feedback from the group. In other words, they do not allow the group to participate in the decision to leave. Such an approach is not calculated to get sincere and meaningful feedback. Members rightfully feel that if the departing member really valued their feedback, he/she would have sought the feedback *before* making the decision. And why shouldn't the group feel that way? After all, the person who decides to leave has been a member of the group for a considerable period of time during which members have come to care about one another and value one another's observations. One would think it only natural that a departing member would *want* to hear what these valued others have to say about the member's wish to terminate. Group members usually feel at first surprised, and later dismissed, disregarded, and hurt by such a cavalier announcement.

The underlying reason for such unilateral terminations is usually not disregard for the group, even though the group may experience that to be the case. More frequently, the departing member has been hurt in one way or another by what has transpired among group members and/or members and the leader, but has not discussed the hurt with the group. Another reason for a unilateral termination is that the person feels unable to withstand the group's scrutiny of the decision without being oppositional or compliant.

Here is an example. Jeanne, a highly valued group member, announced that she has decided to leave the group partly for financial reasons. She stated that she has been in the group for several years, is also in individual therapy, and is about to embark on a 2-month, weekly, cognitive behavioral therapy for which she will be paying out of pocket. She and her husband are in the process of downsizing to pay off large, outstanding credit card bills. She also stated that she has been in therapy for decades and feels she is spending too much time on introspection and not enough time on just living. She also cited an occurrence in the group that made her feel uncomfortable. After having been away for 2 weeks on her vacation and then 3 weeks for the leader's vacation, she felt she was slapped in the face when upon returning the leader announced her unpaid bill (the fact that the bill was 3 months overdue was not announced).

The group brought up several points in discussing the member's intention to leave. If she was trying to save money, why was she opting for a therapy where she had to pay out of pocket for an individual therapy that was much more expensive than group therapy? And why did she think that cognitive therapy would be more helpful than the impressive work she had accomplished in the group? Didn't the fact that the leader owned the fact that he could have waited a week to make the announcement of the unpaid bill, that he had apologized for any undue distress he might have caused, and had said that he would look into why he had made that error—didn't all of those responses make any difference to her? Most of these issues deal with externals.

After the group finished its processing, I said, "It is at times like this that I'm so grateful for our group contract." This statement alerted the group to the fact that Jeanne—by simply announcing that she was planning to leave the group—was not allowing the group to participate in her decision to leave. New material emerged after my remark, which didn't surprise me. A group's failure to comment on a member's not abiding by an item in the contract that everyone initially agreed upon often indicates resistance to certain material. The material being resisted isn't always obvious until it emerges in the group discussion of the contract violation.

As the avoided material came to the surface, I realized that there was resistance to talking about two distinct subjects. One had to do with the group's strong preference not to have to deal with a long-standing competition and antagonism between Jeanne and Margaret that would be revived if extensive attention were given to Jeanne. The other issue involved an emotional injury that Jeanne had sustained in the group that had not previously been acknowledged. It is important to note that the avoided material dealt with deeper issues than those that Jeanne had initially cited for terminating.

The long-standing competitive antagonism concerned which person was the most loathsome and abused member of the group. Jeanne and Margaret vied actively for the title. Each was impressive in her resistance to taking in any of the group's support, acceptance, and caring. The group feared that as it focused on Jeanne's injury in the group, Margaret would once again trot out her well-worn suffering that often led to her chronic suicidal threats. The group wanted to avoid feeling its seeming powerlessness to have any impact on this dynamic.

As the group's concern over the competition was discussed and its fear detoxified, Jeanne felt safe enough to mention an event that had occurred two weeks previously that had played a part in her decision to leave the group. The incident involved another violation of the group contract that had been discussed in the previous two weeks. Audrey had invited Cindy, another group member, to attend a play. Both Audrey and Cindy—abiding by the contract—brought that boundary violation back into the group where the group thought it had been thoroughly discussed, but, as it turned out, not to Jeanne's satisfaction. Jeanne, for the first time, said that she was very hurt that Audrey had not invited *her*. This disclosure reminded the group of Jeanne's history of feeling unwanted, excluded from peer groups in high school and college, and selected last for sports teams. As several group members said they understood how Jeanne could have been hurt by not being invited by Audrey, Jeanne began to tear up.

Jeanne responded to the group's caring and understanding. Group members said they wished there was some way they could help her see and own her many wonderful qualities. The group then commented on how much they thought Jeanne and Margaret had in common. When asked if she was learning something about herself as she watched the group work with Jeanne, Margaret talked about how she too found it hard to believe that other people could see anything of value in her.

This discussion and many others like it helped Jeanne and Margaret become more allies than competitors. Their softened relationship enabled the group to feel safer and do impressive work. Jeanne stayed in the group for two more years. She terminated in a way that included the group in her decision.

Both Jeanne and the group participated in a contract violation. Jeanne announced a unilateral decision to terminate, and the group failed to remind her that she should have discussed the issue in the group *before* making a decision, as stipulated in the contract she had agreed to. An important violation threatened to go undiscussed, an avoidance that would have been harmful to group integrity. My comment, "It is at times like this that I'm grateful for our group contract," facilitated the emergence and discussion of difficult emotional issues that the group, in the end, was able to deal with productively.

Chapter 18

Encouraging the use of imagination

"I don't object to answering that question. I'm simply concerned that in doing so we might value my answers more than your imagination."

A basic assumption here is that imagination is one of the most vital parts of a person. Inviting patients to use their imagination is a way of advancing the treatment and helping them achieve a more substantial self. The way patients respond to such an invitation can have diagnostic and prognostic significance. Some patients, usually those whose early lives have been characterized by severe neglect and/or abuse, have stunted imaginative capacity and limited ability to benefit from exploratory therapy. If and when they are able to develop and utilize imagination—which often takes years of therapy—depends partly on the therapist's belief in the value of imagination.

The importance of imagination in therapy—not to mention in life—was driven home to me during my three-year analysis. In the late 1960s and early 1970s when I was in analysis, analysts did not say a lot during sessions. My analyst had perfected this approach and her relative silence permitted my imagination to roam freely. In my first year of analysis, I somehow had the fantasy that she was having an affair with Eric Erickson. Of course, she said nothing in response to my fantasy and it was not mentioned again. In the third year of analysis, with my imagination already in full swing, I thought she might be having an affair with a senior analyst whose wife had died the year before. In one of her infrequent comments, she replied in her Viennese accent (showing a sense of humor I never knew she had), "Vhat, me be unfaithful to Eric!"

An avid tennis player, my imagination ramped up when a few weeks later she greeted me in the waiting room with her right elbow wrapped in an elastic bandage. I began the session with an excited question, "Are you a tennis player?" to which she replied, "Vell Dr Gans, ve have 50 minutes to explore your associations." What followed was a productive session in which I was given time and space to imagine. What would it be like to play tennis with my analyst? How badly had analysis toned down my competitive instincts? Maybe I had become a less intense person but would I ever again be able to beat an opponent on the court? What would it feel like to defeat her in a match or, even more upsetting,

DOI: 10.4324/9781003174608-22

to lose to a woman 30 years my senior? Would she call the lines fairly—and would I? My analyst, unusually talkative this session, wasted no time making connections between my concern about the fairness of her line calls with some of my father's questionable business practices. In retrospect—she died three years later—I thought that she could have asked me if her elastic bandage stirred up fantasies unrelated to tennis like, for example, the state of her health.

I answer questions only when I think that doing so will advance the work of therapy. When it appears that group members value my answers more than whatever prompted them to ask the question, I appeal to their imaginations. I want to reinforce my conviction that more good will accrue to the therapy from self-reflection than from any answer I can give. One reason for this belief is that some fantasies, products of one's imagination, are very shameful for some people to talk about because we can imagine things that we would never do in real life. Talking to a trusted other can serve to detoxify these fantasies and turn them into just another thought.

At the same time, it is important for therapists to "trust their gut" and answer a question when it feels like the right thing to do. One example of such an indication might be when, after an intense emotional interaction between patient and therapist, the patient asks the therapist "How did you experience me in that interaction?" or "How did my revealing that shameful secret affect your feelings toward me?" Since we do therapy *with* the patient, not to, on, or for the patient, we can always ask when pressed for an answer, "Do you think it would be in your best interest for me to answer this question or should we look into what prompted you to ask?" I try not to say, "Do you think it would be in your best interest for me to answer this question *now*?" I don't want to imply a promise in case exploration of the question indicates it would not be helpful to answer it. It can be flattering to therapists when patients so highly value answers from us. Colluding in that fantasy is often more for the therapist's self-regard than for the patient's benefit.

Many situations in therapy that appear unbidden are grist for the imaginative mill. One morning I felt like I was developing a cold, but as the day went on I felt better and decided not to cancel my evening psychotherapy group. However, once in the group I started to feel a chill and sneezed several times. Joe asked me if I was sick. I encouraged the group to stay with Joe's question. This group had had a stable membership for several years and expected I would invite their thoughts, feelings, and imaginings if or before I answered the question. Esther, who often served as my protector, said that she sometimes went to work when she felt sick even though she knew it was better to stay home. She imagined that I did the same thing. Melvin, who was generally suspicious of other people's motives, was less charitable. He wondered if I had considered the possibility that I could infect members of the group and, if I had, why had I decided to hold the session. Ellen, from a rigid Catholic family, noted that I had just returned from a 3-week vacation and was probably feeling too guilty to cancel the session. George, a hard-driving businessman, wondered why we were spending so much time on this topic. His answer was clear and simple: "You didn't want to lose the money if we didn't meet." After processing their responses (that were so in character), I asked if they wanted an answer to Joe's question. Only George and Melvin wanted me to answer, but they deferred to the members of the group who had an opposite preference and who felt they could learn more from their imaginings than from my answer. I did tell them eventually that I thought it would have been better if I had cancelled the session and that I hoped I had not infected anyone.

Back in the early 1980s one of my mother's brothers who lived in Rochester, New York, died a couple of years after having a bad stroke. He was a superb businessman who made a lot of money and happened to have a white Cadillac that he had bought 6 months before the stroke. I was his favorite nephew and, upon his death, my aunt sold me the car, although I think my uncle would have wanted her to give it to me. Externally, the car was in excellent condition, but as we were to learn over the next year—this was the first year that Cadillac had come out with fuel injection—the car was a lemon, which died going up a hill on a family trip hours from home.

I drove the car from Rochester to Wellesley where I parked it in the driveway of my home where I have an office. My group patients commented on the car the first week it was in the driveway. Seeing the New York State plates, they said that it was nice that we were having company. During the following week, they thought our guests—who they now decided must be relatives—might be overstaying their welcome. By the third week it dawned on them that the Cadillac might actually be mine. They wanted to know if that was so. I invited them to use their imagination. One patient said he had never thought of me as a capitalist pig but that maybe I was one. A second member concluded that I had inherited the car from a recently deceased family member and wondered if the person was someone I had been close to. Was that true, she wanted to know? There was speculation about how much wealth I came from. Another member commented that it had been a long time since I had increased my group rate. He decided that I really didn't need the money, confirming his previous belief that I was living a life of privilege. Whether I had been given the car or had to buy it served as an interesting projective test for the various group members. Not receiving an answer, they suddenly addressed a topic that had been conspicuously avoided in the group: economic disparities among its members. It turned out that one member of the group, who, to the group's surprise, was quite wealthy, felt both guilty in hearing about some members' economic struggles and, as a result, unentitled to bring his issues, which he felt were trivial by comparison, into the group. A subgroup of women mentioned their envy of one woman's stylish and expensive clothing. To the group's titillation, and seemingly out of nowhere, one group member described how she once had screwed up her courage and actually touched the side of my house. "Vinyl siding," she announced to the group's apparent satisfaction and delight. Animation and excitement reigned as my privileged life was brought down a peg.

My decision to retire in June of 2019 stimulated a host of fantasies. At the time I had 3 psychodynamically oriented out-patient psychotherapy groups, each with 8 or 9 members. I thought it would be too emotionally taxing for me to end all three groups at once, so I decided I would end them serially at 6-month intervals. I had to decide which group I would end with first, second, and then last. Each group asked me if they would be the last group to be ended, and I answered their questions. Not surprisingly, the first (A) and second (B) groups I terminated with wanted to know why they weren't the last (C) group I would terminate. As usual, I asked for their associations and fantasies. One member each for groups A and B who had been difficult patients imagined that they were the reason why I was terminating their groups early. Another patient, who had worked through some interpersonally debilitating issues in her 8 years in the group, said that it didn't matter to her in which order I terminated the groups because she had worked hard and received a lot of help from the group and from me. She imagined that I wanted more time to be with the many grand-children she imagined I had. Another person concluded from noticing the work I was having done on my home—I had a home office—that I was fixing up the house to sell it and move to Florida. Another patient, who suffered from low self-esteem, guiltily admitted that she had Googled me. She concluded from my many publications that I cared more about writing papers than seeing patients like her. The group that I ended with last was sure that they were my favorites. They wondered if I had loved my groups (I'm not sure how many they thought I had) equally. Borrowing from the novelist Jane Smiley,[1] I told them "no, that I had loved them individually," an answer that surprisingly seemed to satisfy every member of the group.

Despite the therapeutic value of not answering questions, it is good to remember that there are some situations in which it is important to answer patients' questions. For example, some patients insist that their therapists give them advice. Rather than getting in a struggle with such folks, the therapist can say, "If I were in your situation I might do X, but it is you, not I, that will have to live with that decision and its consequences. What do you imagine the consequences might be?" While giving this reply, I'm mindful of the quote about giving advice: "Advice is a doubtful remedy but seldom harmful because rarely heeded!" Sometimes even relatively healthy people need their questions answered. Mary, one of my group patients and an accomplished businesswoman, said to me, "Dr. Gans, I don't know what you expect to achieve with me by answering my questions with a question. I feel so disrespected by that approach that I shut down internally." Supervised by her feedback, I began answering her questions while, at the same time, worrying that this precedent would lead other group patients to insist that I answer their questions as well. This never happened. The rest of the group appreciated that Mary had this need and seemed relieved that I understood. It was a surprising revelation to me that what I formerly had hoped to achieve with Mary by not answering her questions—greater self-reflection—blossomed with my altered approach.

"Reality is very obliging. You can always count on it to serve up something to complain about. But you can choose how you will respond."

People with character disorders are usually not bothered by the way they are. How they behave does not appear to them to be a matter of choice. They behave the way they do because in their words, "That's just the way I am," even though their behavior is often problematic for other people. They rarely elect psychotherapy on their own. When it seems indicated, they are strongly encouraged by friends to seek out psychotherapy or are brought by family to a psychotherapist when they decompensate.

This chapter focuses on several features of the "chronic complainer." Examples include their tendency to alienate people; the submergence in adulthood of their childhood pain and sadness; their psychodynamics; and the long-term treatment necessary to produce change. Change is possible when they are emotionally ready to accept that they have a choice in how they respond to life's vicissitudes. The therapist's statement "Reality is very obliging. You can always count on it to serve up something to complain about. But you can choose how you will respond" serves to catalyze that awareness.

In the beginning of the movie "Analyze This," Billy Crystal is a psychologist treating a complaining housewife. He tries hard to look interested and empathic but he is bored, frustrated, and annoyed. The movie reverts to an imagined outburst by Crystal where he basically tells her to shut up, get over it, and stop complaining. Therapists who have been inundated with chronic and relentless complaints can identify with Crystal's cathartic eruption.

Emotional pain in the adult character disordered person has been consigned to the deep recesses of their being, in a place that it is not apparent to other people. But their off-putting behaviors are front and center. Their rigidity, control issues, self-absorption, grandiosity, suspiciousness, or stable instability—and, as this chapter highlights, their chronic complaining—repel rather than attract others over the long term. While they seem inured to recurrent rejection and suffering, that impression is not borne out in long-term psychotherapy. It takes a long time in psychotherapy, however, to unearth their anguish and achieve even modest gains. *The gains seem to appear when they come to accept the notion that they have a choice in how they decide to behave.* The teacher appears when the student is ready.

The psychodynamics of chronic complaining provide the therapist with an understanding of this seemingly intractable trait. Persistent complaints can be thought of as transitional objects that are present every morning when the patient wakes up. Stuffed animal equivalents, they are familiar, comforting, and reliable. Chronic complainers don't feel that their complaining is a choice any more than they would think of their heartbeats or respirations as a choice. Complaining is simply what they do, it is ego-syntonic, they are not troubled by it—and often are not particularly concerned or aware that others are. The complaining serves a vital function in the chronic complainer's sense of equilibrium and self-regulation. Chronic complaining is a whine equivalent, a pathetic but annoying whimper to an unresponsive other. It originates early in life when important caretakers are indifferent or harmful.

A personal experience reminded me of the early origins and debilitating effects of whining. I was invited to speak to my daughter's third grade class about what I do as a psychiatrist. After my talk, the teacher asked if anyone had a question for me. Emily, a girl in the back of the room, raised her hand and said, "Dr. Gans, can you help me? I am very, very sad. I don't have any friends and I'm very lonely. I wish I had friends to play with." There was a long, uncomfortable silence. As I was about to say something that I hoped would be comforting, she continued, "And I whine a lot, too." Emily's sadness and emotional pain were palpable and, as the (defensive) laughter in the room indicated, too difficult for her young class-mates to bear.

Adult chronic complainers have a different feel to them. While the sadness in the very young complainer is so apparent, there is little evidence of that pain in the adult chronic complainer. A series of interpersonal failures over time and the hurt and aloneness that result from them calcifies the complaining into a permanent personality trait. The difficult and long-term work in the psychotherapy of adult chronic complainers—and most patients with personality disorders—involves getting beneath their annoying superficial presentation and accessing the emo-tional distress that resides underneath.

Here is a case example. Victoria had no difficulty speaking in the psycho-therapy group that she had recently joined. She took, and the group allowed her to take, a generous amount of time to describe recent and remote hurtful expe-riences. Despite ample airtime, she complained that other people in the group got the lion's share of attention. When the leader—to decrease Victoria's sense of aloneness—gave other group members the opportunity to join her by sharing similar trials in their lives, she complained that the leader was shutting her down. Other members valued her ability to risk unpopularity by speaking truths that catalyzed group work. She could not take in their appreciative comments. She continued to complain that no one in the group liked her—which wasn't true.

The group suggested and Victoria and I agreed that adding individual therapy with me to her group therapy would be useful. A fantasy that I had about Victoria in our group work alerted me to the fact that the exploratory work I was doing with her in individual therapy was not helping.[2] I found myself picturing her com-ing home from school to an empty house, looking sad and lonely. Changing my approach, I tried to become the equivalent of a mother ready with (metaphorical) milk and cookies when she returned from school, eager to hear about her day. She responded to my new way of being with her. Sadness replaced defensiveness as she talked in more detail about the profound deprivation that she experienced early in her life. Gradually she softened. Her complaining markedly decreased. Now in a position where she could be more receptive to understanding and caring, she was able to hear new possibilities opened up by the statement "Reality is very obliging. You can always count on it to serve up something to complain about. But you can choose how you will respond." She began to perceive some things differ-ently. An appreciation of how her boss actually had been supportive in ways she had not previously noticed began to replace her litany of complaints about him.

Instead of expressing disappointment about a series of men that she had dated, she, for the first time, commented that while many of her friends were having major health problems, she hardly ever got sick. She began to take disappointment more in stride, to accept people more for who they were, and, after many years of therapy, to express gratitude for our work together.

My work with Victoria highlights the importance of therapists having and accessing fantasies about their patients. Looking back on the therapy, I realize that I was complaining (to myself) about Victoria's unresponsiveness to my analytic approach. The fantasy of her as a sad little girl coming home to an empty house provided access to a part of her that had escaped my less playful approach. Perhaps I had internalized her complaining mode from which fantasy provided an alternate and more productive approach.

Victoria was the last patient I terminated with before my retirement in June 2019. As I now look back, my pursuing an approach no longer suited to her emotional needs hampered a portion of her treatment. Being responsive to my imagination helped me rectify my mistake. In doing so, I put into practice one of the major lessons about psychotherapy I took from my psychiatric residency training some 48 years ago: be constantly aware of how you might be impeding the very therapeutic enterprise you are trying to advance. I remain indebted to a profession that has required such constant self-scrutiny and honesty.

Notes

1 Smiley, J. (2016). *Early Warning*. New York: Anchor Books, p. 476.
2 Winnicott, D. W. (1971). *Reality and Playing*. New York: Basic Books.

Chapter 19

Welcoming and deepening the negative side of ambivalence

"There are not that many ways to get attention. You can be really, really good or really, really bad."

Childhood is fertile ground for confirming this statement. For some unfathomable reason, a 6-year-old girl is supposed to fully love her newly arrived sibling. Photographs of those early days reveal the truth. The dethroned princess looks forlorn and bereft in the midst of family members oohing and aahing over the new infant. How many stories are there of children packing their little suitcases, threatening to leave home, walking around the block, then returning home, their feeble gesture expressing a sense of cosmic unfairness?

Inequities such as these are as deep as they are forgotten. But the feelings connected to these extreme events in childhood live on in the unconscious until therapy, life experiences, or having children of one's own revive them. These "slings and arrows of outrageous fortune" penetrate so deeply that the afflicted only know that they hurt while not knowing why. Surely, the ill-timed arrival of a sibling could not account for a lifetime of unhappiness, envy, rage, or depression. Or could it? Therapists have no shortage of patients who feel that they got a raw deal when a sibling was born and they were suddenly overlooked and felt invisible.

A patient of mine had two sons, one a relentless and impressive achiever, the other an incorrigible slacker and troublemaker. His "good son" resented the "bad son" for the amount of family attention he received. The father decided to institute an award system, hoping that the points and the related rewards that his "bad" son received would encourage him to do better in school and select more appropriate friends. At the end of the first month the "good" son had amassed 104 points, the "bad" son 11. They each, apparently, had staked out their respective territory.

What is counterintuitive in this scenario is that just as much suffering can exist in the "very, very good" child as exists in the "very, very bad" child. The "good" child may become an achievement addict or a compulsive people-pleaser at the expense of accessing and expressing authentic feelings, especially the so-called negative ones. Some of these folks show up in their therapists' offices in their late twenties or early thirties not knowing about their dark side. They aren't aware of

DOI: 10.4324/9781003174608-23

ever having experienced envy, sadism, Schadenfreude, vengeance, or hate. They develop what Winnicott has called the False Self.[1]

A variety of developmental dynamics contribute to this outcome. Some folks, as Alain De Botton points out in his book, *The Course of Love*, grow up to understand the love of others as a reward for being good.[2] Bad behavior threatens that love. Others feel the compulsion to be good as a way of defending against the dim awareness of anger at parents who have greatly disappointed them. Still others may have the misfortune of having a disruptive sibling who makes family life miserable. Taking care of their parents, especially ones who are fragile, seems the least they can do, especially when they sense there is no parental objection.

Many people have a need to appear flawless or invulnerable to criticism. Recently I treated a couple where the woman had impressive academic credentials and prided herself on being an "independent, professional woman." She then related the following marital grievance. She complained that her husband would often make disparaging remarks about some of her choices and gave the following example. While in the voting booth with her 10-year-old son, she realized that she was reluctant to vote for a Democratic candidate for fear that her son would tell her husband about her choice, and that he would disapprove. In a subsequent marital session, her husband contended that this story revealed much more about his wife's need to please than any of his expectations or comments. With another patient, I came to expect that she would continue to pick the dead leaves off my waiting room plants, hoping for my love in return. A third patient would, without fail, pay her bill immediately upon receiving it, even though my policy is that I bill at the end of the month and expect payment within a month. The handwriting on the check was flawless.

It is impressive when such goodie-goodies begin to let loose in therapy. On one occasion I went into the waiting room to receive a very compliant patient who happened to be reading a magazine that appeared to engage him. I could tell that even though he resented being interrupted, he entered the office and politely began his story. As is occasionally my wont, and since the timing seemed right, I began a soliloquy while looking out the window and speaking to no one in particular. The purpose of the soliloquy was to capture what I thought the patient was really thinking and feeling but not revealing. I said: "Psychotherapy is really a lot crap. I mean, how long does it take to get better and, for that matter, how do you actually know if you have changed at all? And my therapist just sits there and hardly talks."

Before I realized, the patient got up out of his chair, went over to my fish tank and said, "What a stupid hobby." He then went over to two prints hanging on my office wall that had women with indistinct faces and said, "Just like a psychiatrist, everything is a God damn Rorschach test, you couldn't have a person with a normal face, could you?" I began to think about my homeowners insurance as he picked up a ceramic vase that I was afraid he was going to throw through a window or at me. As he continued to walk around the office, he seemed for the first time ever to be relaxed, unlike his usual robotic self. He then proceeded to tell me that his mother weighed over 300 pounds and that at the dinner table one had to raise one's hand and be called on before speaking, disclosures he had never made before in his weekly, 3-year therapy.

Therapists need to be careful not to exploit "the relatively easy therapeutic hour" that such very good patients offer us. Given the emotionally consuming stories that we listen to hour after hour, day after day, we may unconsciously welcome the respite that such very, very good patients provide. I was alerted to this phenomenon during a group therapy session in which I noticed how very much I was missing Natalie, a patient who was on vacation. Natalie was the consummate diplomat, an expert at calming troubled waters. My stomach dropped as I realized for the first time the extent to which I had counted on her reasonableness to bribe other group members out of their difficult to deal with feelings. I reminded myself that she was in the group because of her own pain and suffering and vowed to do better by her—and the group—in the future. It was probably because of her excessive niceness that I wanted to avoid being a casualty when the "bomb" undoubtedly buried inside of her detonated. It is very easy for us to forget that often in our very, very good patients there resides just as much emotional pain as exists in our very, very bad patients.

Growing up, very, very good people have never been introduced to their negative feelings. It has been a matter of survival for them not to know of the existence in them of feelings such as anger, hostility, sadism, hate, and vengeance. The cost of this estrangement has been the absence of the gradual civilizing that results from exposure to such feelings over time. What has never developed is the ability to modulate and regulate the expression of such feelings. Instead, their eruption in adulthood is like trying to get a drink from a fire hose. Picture the person trying to get such a drink: head snapped back, body thrown to the ground, and swept away supine by the force of the water. It is no wonder in treating such people in psychotherapy that therapists are invested, often unwittingly, in not wanting to tamper with the patient's niceness. They prefer not to be in the line of fire when seemingly out of nowhere such negative feelings erupt.

To patients who accuse me of not caring about them, I DON'T say "It *feels* to you that you have an uncaring therapist." Instead, I say, "What is it like for you to have an uncaring therapist?"

Psychotherapy patients have many prerogatives. They can deny, distort, and project. They can accuse their therapists of not caring or doing a lousy job. They can blame their therapists for *their own* shortcomings. They can accuse their therapists of only being interested in taking their money. Psychotherapy patients have also a few responsibilities: they (eventually) need to work on their feelings and accusations rather than simply indulge them, and they must pay for their therapy in a timely fashion.

Protected in part by their therapeutic role and their awareness that such comments are coming from people whose problems have caused them to seek help, therapists are able not to take such comments personally (although when therapists realize that these accusations have merit, they need to respond honestly to them). Sitting, hour after hour, listening to such material combined with something amiss in their personal lives can cause such attacks to break through therapists' defenses. When this happens, self-protection can take precedence over caring for the patient.

Therapists' efforts to protect themselves run the spectrum. At one end of the spectrum, therapists dispose of such patients—as in making a disposition. Some therapists are not cut out—or prefer not—to work with such patients. Referring these patients may be a sign of maturity and indicate an ability to acknowledge limitation. At the other end of the spectrum, therapists who have actually terminated such patients psychologically continue to treat them. An honest acknowledgment of a lack of chemistry with the patient would have better served both. Midway between the ends of the spectrum, therapists minimize patients' feelings or do not take them seriously. They do this by suggesting that what their patients are feeling about their therapists—that they are deficient, inept, uncaring—is subjective and has no real basis in reality. The patient merely feels this way.

The comment "What is it like for you to have an uncaring therapist?" strives for the opposite effect: to confirm, even deepen, the patient's feeling. The therapist does not make this statement because she believes it is true. The therapist employs it to make it clear that she notices, understands, accepts, and validates that the patient feels this way.

This comment frequently has several effects:

1   The patient feels heard.
2   The patient realizes that he does not need to keep making these feelings known, the therapist "gets it."
3   Since the patient expects the other person to defend him/herself, the patient is temporarily thrown off balance when this doesn't happen.
4   The patient now has the opportunity to realize gradually that the "action" is temporarily no longer between him and his therapist but, rather, between him and himself. In effect, the therapist has conveyed, "Given that you come every week to a therapist who doesn't care about you, how do you think about proceeding?"
5   At this juncture the patient can leave therapy, explore his feelings about leaving therapy, or look inward and deepen the therapeutic work.
6   If the patient seriously entertains the option of leaving the therapy, and if the therapy has really been important and meaningful to the patient, the denied positive side of the patient's ambivalence either asserts itself or becomes more difficult to deny.
7   If the patient decides to stay in therapy, the focus tends to shift from blame to introspection.

Earlier in my career I was reluctant to offer the comment "What is it like for you to have an uncaring therapist?" for fear that it would confirm the patient's negative experience of me. In the vast majority of cases this is not what happened. What I imagine transpired in the patient was reassurance that even when under attack I was still able to be empathic to his/her experience. Such a therapeutic stance is to be differentiated from a therapist's masochistic submission to repeated, unremitting, gratuitous attacks—a behavior that the patient has shown no interest in or intention of working on over a prolonged period of time.

It is important to note that the statement "What is it like for you to have an uncaring therapist?" does not advance the therapy with all patients, especially those with major attachment disorders. People with a reduced capacity for, and a pervasive pattern of detachment from, social relationships may denigrate their therapists as a (dysfunctional) way of maintaining needed distance. They can't tolerate intense feelings and are more comfortable with solitary activities. Their suspiciousness and vulnerability to perceived rejection may cause them to mistake their therapist's curiosity and empathy for mockery. On the other hand, such a formulation assumes that such traits are fixed and unalterable, a view that is at odds with the currently accepted idea that what transpires in psychotherapy is co-constructed. I have treated in long-term therapy several character-disordered patients who had a limited capacity for intimacy. While the changes they made have been modest, these modest changes have made a significant difference in their ability to have closer emotional relationships. The question "What is it like for you to have an uncaring therapist?" has allowed them over many years to express and soften their negative feelings. With their venom dissipated, their projections are less liable to make other people seem unapproachable.

Recall the contrast after a severe blizzard when, the following day, brilliant sunshine fills the sky. Something akin to that dramatic change occurs in the therapy after the patient has had the opportunity to vent spleen over a long period of time. At some level, even if never put into words, the patient realizes that his therapist has been understanding, invested, curious, non-judgmental, unflappable, and non-retaliatory even when made the object of hateful feelings (meant for someone else). The patient senses that his therapist understands the apprehension, the deliberation, the need, the vulnerability, the courage, and the relief that have accompanied his diatribes. Over time and with many repetitions, the patient comes to realize that his therapist grasps the importance of "my need to get these feelings out" and the therapeutic benefits that often result from doing so. The "good mom" of the very difficult adolescent may wait decades until her now grown child acknowledges his good fortune at having had such an understanding, accepting, and mature parent. One of the fringe benefits of our profession is the expression of gratitude that often accompanies the final stages of a therapy that follows the path described earlier.

Notes

1 Winnicott, D. W. (1971). *Reality and Playing*. New York: Basic Books.
2 De Botton, A. (2017). *The Course of Love*. New York: Simon & Schuster, p. 74.

Chapter 20

Employing methods of the Existential School of psychiatry

"What do you want me to be sure to hear when you tell me that a comment of mine makes you uncomfortable?"

In several consecutive sessions of a T-group I led for first-year psychiatric residents, they directed a lot of criticism at the administration and at their residency training director. I said something about their criticising that upset them. Several residents complained that my comment made them feel uncomfortable. I responded, "What do you want me to be sure to hear when you tell me that a comment of mine makes you uncomfortable?" I think what they wanted to say was "Fuck you, we're already overloaded and overwhelmed with the pain of our psychotic and decompensated character disordered patients; we don't need anymore." Clearly, administration and the residency training director were safer targets—especially at a distance. (It's worth noting that generally in a 3-year T-group there is a different and predictable target each year for the residents' dissatisfaction: In the first year it's the administration; in the second year, the T-group leader, and in the third year, each other. There is greater valuing of each other in the third year as well.)

They ignored my comment until one resident said to a disgruntled fellow resident, "He's got a point. What if you were the residency director for a surgical training program and a candidate for the program said that he was very motivated to become a surgeon but couldn't stand the sight of blood?" In an attempt to amplify my question, I asked: "How will you ever be able to forgive these patients for making you get in touch with parts of you that, up to this point in your lives, you have had the luxury of not noticing?" Here I was referring to feelings such as hatred, sadism, powerlessness, intolerable loneliness, extreme stubbornness, overwhelming sexual attraction, unworkable passivity, profound dependency, psychotic depression, and rage.

As I think back, I realize that early in my career I shared some of those same concerns. Two years out of residency training I was a staff psychiatrist at a mental hospital. Evelyn, a very attractive 33-year-old woman suffering from a major depression, was admitted to the hospital and became my patient. She gradually emerged from her depression with a compelling radiance and began to express

DOI: 10.4324/9781003174608-24

warm feelings for me. For a short period of time, it wasn't clear if she was recovering from her depression or slowly converting to mania. At the time, I was 34, had been married for 9 years, and had a one-year-old daughter. When the patient called a florist and had rose petals scattered on the driveway of the mental hospital as a sign of her love and urged me to consummate the relationship in a nearby hotel, it became clear that more than a healthy recovery from depression was taking place. As Evelyn's mental condition did escalate to mania, I quickly reality tested her feelings for me by telling her that I was happily married and available only as her therapist. Shortly after making that comment, I realized that I was so threatened by the sexual feelings that Evelyn stirred up in me that what I said to her was as much or more for my benefit than it was for hers.

I have found the Existential School of psychiatry has much to teach us about patients who cause us to deal with our difficult and unacceptable feelings (See Chapter 21 for a discussion of patients whose emotional pain makes them difficult to sit with.).[1] Its methods serve to clear the therapeutic field of labels. In existential therapy, clinicians can't take solace in descriptors: you are the patient, I am the therapist; you are sick, I am healthy; I know better than you do what is good for you; I possess the truth, you do not. Granted, the person who comes for help is a patient—and pays for a service—but the therapist makes every effort not to approach the treatment in the traditional manner. The major effect of this approach has been to help me be emotionally present rather than smart, correct, insightful, or to feel superior and in control. It taught me that with sicker patients especially, these attributes were not helpful.

The Existential School of psychiatry starts with the premise that the truth is impossible to completely establish and that insight is of limited value to very emotionally troubled people. We can't take comfort in the notion that the "truth will make you free" because the truth is unattainable. It can only be approximated. Nor has the therapist cornered the market on the best way to live. What is thought to be helpful to people who feel like untouchables are the therapist's determination to *approximate* being and staying with where the patient is emotionally. This determination is thought to be therapeutic because such patients know very well, through experience, that others find them difficult to be with and, as a consequence, avoid or even shun them.

The effort, the caring, and the willingness to endure the feelings of powerlessness, helplessness, attraction, superiority, rage, frustration, and even disgust that these patients evoke slowly sends a message that no other approach has achieved: *I am here, dedicated to trying to be and stay with your feelings*. The uniqueness of that experience for the patient is considered to be an important therapeutic ingredient because the patient has had little to no experience with a caring other who is so determined and dedicated. At some level, the patient grasps the fact that the helper is bearing great discomfort in the service of staying with a very troubled and troubling other. In exchange for such thrusting of oneself into the emotional experience of the other, the therapist is relieved of the burden of being smart or being right.

The concept of "successive approximation" is related to the collaborative pursuit of emotional truth rather than the therapist's efforts to cognitively understand. In the employment of successive approximation, it doesn't matter who brings the dyad closer to a never fully apprehended emotional truth. If the patient (for lack of a better designation) is more effective in this step-by-step pursuit, the helper is delighted. If the helper hits the mark, it becomes clear the patient feels profoundly joined.

A 40-year-old internist, from a prominent family, was recovering from a major depression. He described what took place on his December 23rd birthday when he was a latency-aged child. His mother took him and his invited friends on a hired bus to a poor section of town where his birthday gifts were distributed to poor children for Christmas. He was expected to be happy as his gifts were given out. In the therapy, for the first time in his life, he was getting in touch with the profound deprivation involved. His therapist, accessing his visceral response to the story and successively approximating emotional truth, said, "It's enough to make one sick to one's stomach." The internist began sobbing uncontrollably.

A more traditional psychodynamic approach might have invited the patient to remember other incidents where his mother was tone deaf to childhood feelings he had experienced.

****

Back to T-group. My hope in running the T-group was not to train a cadre of psychiatrists who would necessarily choose to treat very sick patients. My goal was to help them to become more aware, even with less sick patients, of disturbing feelings that are often present in any clinical encounter. The question, "What do you want me to be sure to hear when you tell me that a comment of mine makes you uncomfortable?" was meant to serve two *eventual* purposes. The first was to help these first-year residents deal with, not avoid or blame others for the difficult feelings stirred up in them by their patients. The second was to help them realize that in processing their own feelings they would be in a better position to respond to their patients therapeutically. These skills are an essential part of becoming a psychiatrist.

"What is it like coming every week to a therapist who doesn't answer your questions, repeatedly misses the mark with her comments, and isn't helping you?"

What therapist has not had the experience of looking at her appointment book, seeing that the next patient is Henry, and then dreading the appointment? For weeks if not months, Henry has been directing at his therapist a barrage of disappointments, demands, threats to leave the treatment, and attacks on the therapist's competence or caring. These remarks begin to take their toll. Nothing the therapist says is useful or comforting. The therapist takes a step back and wonders if she and the patient are working at cross-purposes. She is expecting a patient capable of and interested in emotional exploration. Her patient subscribes to the carwash theory of psychotherapy—show up, receive soap and water, wax, and drying, and come off the therapeutic conveyor belt feeling much better. The therapist decides to give the patient the benefit of the doubt and to keep working with him. But over time nothing seems to change. (All these considerations assume that the therapist has been doing a competent job.)

Finally, the therapist decides to reflect on Henry's criticisms to see if there is merit in what he is saying. If that is the case, the therapist needs to take Henry's criticism to heart and look inward. Supervision or therapy for the therapist may be in order.

This relentless battering of the therapist has a timeless quality. It becomes difficult for the therapist to envision a time when the sun will emerge from behind the clouds. The therapist begins to lose sight of what she and the patient initially agreed to work on in the therapy. Somehow the therapist has lost therapeutic leverage; in fact, she finds herself more invested in her patient's therapy than he is. To compound matters, she begins to question her therapeutic skills. She may even be losing sleep at night.

Caught in a projective beam of hostility and disparagement from which there appears to be no escape, the therapist tries harder to connect with the patient. Nothing works. A sado-masochistic dynamic emerges wherein the therapist feels progressively more powerless and demeaned while the patient, who continues to verbally assault the therapist, feels increasingly misunderstood, frustrated, and hopeless. Therapist–patient distance increases.

What is counterintuitive about this scenario is that Henry, who creates distance through relentless disparagement, craves closeness and warmth and, at the same time, can tolerate neither. Further complicating the impasse, Henry is not aware of his predicament.

Attempts to satisfy his cravings diminish his chances of appreciating his dilemma. He continues to believe that a competent therapist would make him feel better. He continues to focus on his therapist's inadequacies rather than to look inward. His therapist's efforts to try harder simply reinforce Henry's belief that the problem exists outside of him. A discouraged, depleted therapist and a frustrated, disappointed, and angry patient have reached a stalemate. At this point, the therapy appears destined to fail.

A possible remedy for this impasse resides in a strategy that strives to move Henry from being mad to being sad. The sadness will result from helping him get in touch with the possibility that he could lose his therapist. The assumption here is that Henry has ambivalent feelings toward his therapist. If he had only negative feelings toward her he would most probably have already left the therapy. His dilemma, presently, is that his positive feelings for his therapist are too threatening for him to access. If he is to be able to tolerate these positive feelings, he will need to be introduced to them gradually. Asking the question "What is it like coming every week to a therapist who doesn't answer your questions, who repeatedly misses the mark with her comments, and who isn't helping you?" attempts to achieve this goal.

The following imagined exchange between Henry and his therapist illustrates how this approach might play out. When his therapist finally asks Henry this question, his thinking could take him in a variety of directions. He could explain why he doesn't feel comfortable with or understood by her. He might say he thinks he would do better with a male therapist. He might say that her brand of therapy is not what he needs. His thoughts might go to the possibility of terminating the therapy.

What might Henry then think or feel when his therapist seems open to talking about that possibility? First, Henry finds it harder to sustain the illusion that his therapist has all the power when it is clear that he does have the option to leave treatment. A hint of the therapist's concern might occur to him as he realizes that she cares enough about him to respect his decision to leave therapy if that is what he feels he needs to do. He notices that his therapist neither tries to talk him out of such a decision nor encourages him to stay. She continues to be interested in exploring his thinking about the decision. It's a slightly new feeling for him to experience his therapist being more interested in his disappointment than in protecting her narcissism. As Henry considers his options, if there are hidden positive feelings toward his therapist, imagining leaving her for good could get him in touch with sad feelings. If he mentions feeling sad or appears sad, a new and different kind of discussion would now be possible.

A focus on the relative perceived size of the patient and therapist is instructive here. It seems likely that Henry, feeling so small, experiences his therapist as so large that he needs to bring her down in size with repeated attacks. His therapist's response surprises him. Rather than getting puffed up with defensiveness, she sadly acknowledges that she has failed him. The sado-masochistic dynamic defused, and with no one left for Henry to attack, he is now freed up to feel fear, loneliness, and maybe a twinge of sadness.

In fact, in this example, if Henry's therapist had not finally made her intervention, she would have been at risk of participating in a masochistic submission to an unrelenting attack—a posture that would have been a disservice to the patient, the therapy, and certainly, his therapist.

Several possible considerations emerge if Henry does not feel anything positive toward his therapist. Maybe she is the wrong therapist for Henry, possibly the chemistry isn't there. Perhaps, for whatever reason, she just doesn't understand Henry or can't relate to him in a way that makes him feel cared about. Perhaps her theoretical orientation requires a degree of cognitive and emotional processing of which Henry is not developmentally capable. Or, is Henry's strongest connection not to other people but to his own perceptions and views of the world, a schizoid orientation? Perhaps Henry's devaluing attitude is a characterological trait that interferes with his ability to take in and feel caring from another person. Instead, he has to settle for the *consolation* prize of being "right"—"if I can't have love, at least I can be right" (in my assessment of my therapist).

It is worth noting that therapists may be reluctant to make a statement that affirms the patient's negative perceptions of them for fear that in doing so the patient's perceptions are confirmed and solidified. That has not been my experience. Rather, the patient usually derives some measure of reassurance from a therapist who, while under unremitting attack, remains empathically tuned in to the patient's pain.

If Henry does decide to terminate therapy, his therapist should comport herself as he leaves in a manner that heightens the chances that Henry would seek therapy in the future should the need arise. A stance characterized by respect for him as well as his decision, non-judgment, caring, and well wishes would go far in reaching this goal.

The reader may have noticed that nowhere in this chapter do I comment on or allude to Henry's past and what he might be reenacting, or where he might have learned (and needed) his combative style. In doing so I have assumed an existential position where the goal is stay with the here-and-now emotional experience of the patient, an approach that differs from traditional psychodynamic technique.

Note

1 Havens, L. (1974). The existential use of the self. *Am J Psychiatry*: 1–10.

Chapter 21

Miscellaneous

Assessing suicidality

> **"If your suicidal feelings were to become more frequent and intense, and you were not sure that you could resist acting on them, what do you imagine you would do?"**

The New York State Board of Regents, which is responsible for the general supervision of all educational activities within the state, had what I thought was a curious oath that students were required to sign at the end of a final exam. Students were required to state that they had not cheated. I could never understand why the Board of Regents would think a student who had cheated on an exam would have a scruple about falsely stating under oath that she had not cheated. (The only rationale that I can think of for having such an oath is the difference between cheating and lying under oath. Cheating is a moral failure while lying under oath is perjury, which is a crime. Even so, most high school students would probably not be aware of this distinction.)

In a similar vein, I have never understood the faith that clinicians in recent times have placed on "contracting for safety" with suicidal patients. In this procedure, suicidal patients agree not to harm themselves over a certain time period. I've wondered "Why would a patient who wanted to take his own life persuade himself to stay alive merely because he had made a promise to a therapist?" Such a promise, it seems to me, provides the therapist with the illusion of safety rather than with safety itself. Were such a contract actually to result in safety, that outcome would, in the majority of cases, have less to do with the agreement and more to do with a competent assessment of the following factors: the state of the therapeutic alliance; the therapist's skill in welcoming into the therapy the most desperate, anguished parts of the patient's thinking; any history of past suicide attempts by the patient, especially in the recent past; the degree of lethality of any previous suicide attempts or gestures the patient had made; the patient's age and degree of social isolation; an existing social support system; and a history of suicide in the patient's family.

DOI: 10.4324/9781003174608-25

Notice that first on my list of suicidal deterrents is the therapeutic alliance. Often, though not always, it is the robustness of the therapeutic alliance and the mutual dedication to the therapeutic work that keeps a patient in the throes of intense suicidal feelings alive. The question—"If your suicidal feelings were to become more frequent and intense, and you were not sure that you could resist acting on them, what do you imagine you would do?"—takes measure of the therapeutic alliance by asking what the patient imagines she would do in the depths of her suicidal anguish. What the therapist is trying to learn here, among other things, is whether the patient would call the therapist or some trusted other. Absent that answer, the therapist would inquire why the patient would not consider calling her—or maybe anyone.

This question assists the therapist in evaluating the possible reasons why the suicidal patient would not make such a call. One possibility is that the patient is determined to kill herself and doesn't want anyone to stop her. If that is the case the therapist welcomes in more of the patient's anguish for exploration and tries to make an alliance with the small part of the patient that does want to live; after all, if 100% of her wanted to die, the patient and therapist would not be having this conversation. If the patient feels that her therapist doesn't really care about her, the reasons for the patient's feeling that way could be discussed. Those reasons could include past behaviors of the therapist, recent disruptions in the patient–therapist relationship, or the patient's sense that her therapist's investment in her professional reputation would take precedence over doing what was best for the patient. If the patient fears that the result of calling her therapist would be immediate hospitalization, they could have a conversation about the possibility of hospitalization in the service of providing temporary and needed safety.

Another reason the patient might not call her therapist or a valued other has to do with the patient's experience around needing help. Did the patient learn early in life that help was not readily available, so don't bother to ask and just learn to figure out things alone? Or that needing help is shameful and "independence" avoids humiliation? Exploring with the patient the limiting and destructive nature of these strategies might help the patient consider healthier ways of proceeding.

All of these conversations convey a powerful meta-communication: "I care about you. I will lend you this caring while you are unable to care about yourself. Your unbearable feelings—which I take seriously—are not overwhelming me and I remain dependably present to be of help. I respect your ultimate decision and know that it is your choice finally to choose life or not." It is this enduring interest in and caring for the patient that is her most precious lifeline.

While proceeding with the inquiries it is important for the therapist to keep in mind, especially with patients determined to kill themselves, that some of these patients may not be telling the truth or may be deliberately withholding critical information. Intuition is not a useful clinical attribute when imminent suicidal intentions are deliberately withheld. Because therapists often pride themselves on their intuitive abilities, they often neglect to keep in the front of their minds the possibility that their suicidal patient may be consciously withholding crucial information.

Treating marital conflict in individual therapy

"How did such a kind, caring woman like you happen to choose a man like Martin?"

Years ago, my in-laws were at a cocktail party where the conversation centered on a man who was not present. The man's job was slaughtering animals according to the rules of Kashrut. (The Yiddish word for this occupation is "shochet.") Those present described him as kind, gentle, compassionate, and extremely loving. The conversation continued in this vein for about 5 minutes until someone interrupted, "Until he happens to be around chickens."

People are complex and have a variety of selves that emerge in various settings and differ depending on a number of variables. A person may present one way in an academic setting, another way in an athletic venue, and still another way with family members. Despite such a collection and range of selves, each person's self-perception is usually narrower and more constricted. Nowhere is this truer than in individual therapy where an unhappily married person speaks of his/her spouse. Usually the patient-spouse appears to have cornered the market on all admirable qualities while the disappointing spouse apparently possesses only negative qualities.

The single-minded version with which the disaffected spouse portrays his/her experience of the marriage can be very convincing. No shades of gray, no complexity, no irony finds its way into the narrative. The certitude of such an account flies in the face of Nature's incredible variety—the plenitude of over 25,000 species of orchids, the broad spectrum of greens found in a mountain landscape, the human microbiome that consists of 100 trillion cells—to mention a few.

It is not surprising that couples in marital therapy have a lower divorce rate than marriages in which only one member of the couple is in therapy. One explanation for this discrepancy is that in marital therapy the therapist hears both sides of the story. The playing field is thereby leveled. When only one member of the couple is in therapy, some therapists have trouble maintaining neutrality or imagining other perspectives, so persuasive is the account of the aggrieved spouse (or so lacking is the training of the therapist).

What is taking place? The unconscious psychological mechanism of projective identification is thought to be at work here.[1] In contrast to the psychological defense mechanism of projection where negative parts of the person are assigned to others who are then avoided, in projective identification disowned parts of the self are experienced to exist in the other *with whom the projector becomes preoccupied, if not vigilant.* Believing that all the negative qualities exist in the other, the projector's job now is to keep his/her eye on this untrustworthy, problematic, impossible-to-satisfy, or possibly dangerous other, and to self-protect. What makes this dynamic so resistant to change, so hard to interrupt, is that people tend to believe their projections so strongly that they are often not amenable to rational persuasion.

The question "How did such a kind, caring woman like you happen to choose a man like Martin?" is designed to impart a benign skepticism to the aggrieved spouse's one-sided account of the other. The usual response, when boiled down to its essence, is that "He wasn't like that when I met him." Admittedly, some individuals can at times be so convincingly deceptive that most people would be taken in and fooled. In the majority of cases, however, there are telltale clues, cautionary signs: recurrent lateness, unprompted mood swings, financial irresponsibility, explanations that don't compute, previous marital infidelity, and estrangement from parents.

Further exploration reveals that covert bargains were made at the beginning of their relationship. The unconscious attractions that led to these agreements fit each other's personality profiles and short-term emotional needs. For example, Martin, a very successful businessman, always tried as a child to please his self-absorbed mother by doing whatever she asked of him. As an adult he dealt with his deep-seated doubts about his self-worth by compulsively providing for others. His wife, Madeleine, grew up with an intermittently psychotic father. She dealt with her childhood demons by imagining that she came from nobility. Their covert, unconscious pre-marital "deal" went something like this: Madeleine. "I'll endorse your compulsive need to give to others (and especially me) if you agree to indulge all my desires and extravagant fantasies." Martin: "If you give me the love I never got from my mother, I'll treat you like royalty." Ultimately, Martin came to feel that he existed merely to service his wife. Madeleine came to believe that while Martin loved the idea of giving, he didn't love her—or know how to love.

With the question "How did such a kind, caring woman like you happen to choose a man like Martin?" the therapist treads on sensitive territory. Up to this point in the therapy, a concerted effort has been made to be supportive of the patient's point of view. The aim has been to join with the patient and empathize with her experience, all in the service of solidifying trust and bolstering the therapeutic alliance. At the same time, the therapist is listening to the material with the knowledge that relationships are co-constructed, that each member is contributing to the form and direction that the relationship assumes.

The patient's reaction to this question, immediately or over time, provides the therapist with important data. The person who responds to the question with curiosity and introspection differs greatly from the one who feels betrayed and suddenly views the therapist with caution and suspicion. In the latter instance, the therapist might get a first taste of what it has been like for the vilified spouse when he attempted to entertain a viewpoint that differed from his wife's. Conversely, the therapist who simply confirms a spouse's version of a conflict-laden marriage confines that person to the status of victim.

Since every therapist has a unique style for approaching blind spots, some might find my question, asked with irony, "How did such a kind, caring woman like you happen to choose a man like him?" needlessly provocative. A perhaps less ironic and more direct approach might be, "Do you feel that you might be contributing anything to the marriage that elicits meaningless and loveless giving by your husband?" (It is worth noting that a gender bias might be at work here. Two women who read the manuscript thought the ironic question was kinder than the question "Do you feel that you might be contributing anything to the marriage that elicits meaningless and loveless giving by your husband?")

Recognizing and acknowledging the emotional pain of patients who are difficult to like and to be with

"We all have our preferences for how pain is gift-wrapped. But, no matter how it is gift wrapped, remember, pain is pain."

We find some patients more likeable and easier to work with than others. Put in other terms, the patients we find more congenial evoke in us feelings that are not problematic, feelings that we are more familiar with. Patients we refer to as difficult are beset by a variety of disruptive feelings. In order to be empathic to these patients, caretakers have to access similar feelings in themselves. Doing so can be uncomfortable or frightening for caretakers who so far in their lives have had the luxury of not dealing with these feelings. (Some emotions, such as hate, are difficult to work with even for caretakers who have experience with these feelings.) It is with these latter two groups of patients that we have the hardest time recognizing and acknowledging their emotional pain. A large part of my first year of psychiatric residency involved that experience.

My work as a liaison psychiatrist in an acute physical rehabilitation hospital highlighted one group of patients that the rehabilitation team found difficult to work with: chronic pain patients. I would often be called to see patients who complained, day after day, that their present pain was worse than their pain the day before. Nothing seemed to help, not medication, not physical therapy, not heat, not cold. Initially responsive, the staff progressively became perplexed, frustrated, disbelieving—"more pain than yesterday, not possible"—and, finally, angry. Their credulity strained, the staff requested a psychiatric consultation.

I assumed a position opposite to the staff's, made possible in part because I wasn't responsible for the day-to-day care of these patients. I wondered with these patients if it was possible that they actually had *more* pain than they contended, not only pain in their bodies but (emotional) pain in their lives. If nothing else, the distinctiveness of my attitude caught their attention. I became the first person who was not implying that the "pain was all in their heads." I seemed to be on their side. In more cases than not, I was correct about something being amiss in their lives. The fact that I wasn't invested in being right about the locus of their pain made it easier for them to consider the relevance of their emotional and social difficulties to the persistence of their physical pain.

When I was able to tell their personal stories, staff attitudes softened. Social service became involved with their families. As this personal information filtered down to the rehabilitation team, understanding and a more compassionate approach replaced what had become a counterproductive judgmental attitude toward the patient.

As a group therapist I tried to pay particular attention to the member who was in the greatest pain in a given session. I also tried to provide safety for the most chronically vulnerable members. They were people whose emotional development lagged behind that of the other group members. Morey was one such patient.

When Morey became anxious in the group, he was sure it was due to insufficient oxygen in the room and asked if he could open a window. When he was afraid he was going to be unable to breathe, he would leave the group and sit in the waiting room until he felt better. The group became impatient with his somatizing, advice-giving, and preoccupation with behavior rather than feeling.

Group members were especially intolerant of what they felt was Morey's superficiality, extreme neediness, and tendency to assume what people were feeling rather than asking them what they were feeling. When they became particularly impatient with him, I would invite them to see what it was *in them*, rather than what it was about Morey, that so upset them. All the group members would work with my question except Esther. She became furious at me when I would continue to invite her to look inside to see what Morey triggered in her.

Summoning up her courage, she confronted me about (what she felt was) a blind spot of mine. She explained that in her individual therapy she was working on her anger at her mentally ill brother who sucked up all the family's attention when she was growing up, leaving her neglected. She said that part of her emotional work was to get out her anger at her brother, and if Morey was the temporary target for that anger so be it. It was not her job to protect Morey and, furthermore, she didn't feel like protecting him because he was repeating for her in group the emotional deprivation she suffered growing up. She also pointed out that my job was *not* to repeat her parents' failure to attend to her needs. And she was right on both counts. When I finally was able to hear what she was telling me, I gave her credit for her courage and perseverance. I apologized for prioritizing Morey's neediness over her suffering. That interaction turned out to be a turning point in Ether's treatment. This experience re-taught me a lesson I thought I already knew: everyone's emotional pain, everyone's subjectivity is real, and matters.

Sometimes it is very difficult for patients who function in the world to identify with severely impaired group members. Martha hadn't worked in years and, during her 20-year stay in the group, had seen many people join and graduate from the group. She conjured up in my mind a fellow student from grammar school and high school who was twice held back and who had no friends. Martha rarely missed a group meeting and seemed to value her connections with other group members. One evening, seemingly out of the blue, she said to the group, "The longer I'm in this group, the more I realize how much I love my dog. And, you know, I don't even have a dog." Group members said they didn't have words for what they just heard. A feeling of profound sadness enveloped the group. A few weeks later when Martha was absent, group members talked about how frightening it was to grasp how emotionally damaged a person could be. Despite their inability to identify with the nature of Martha's impairment, they genuinely gave her credit for the courage it took for her to make it through each day. In Martha's case, they did the hard work of validating a kind of pain they couldn't imagine existing in their own lives.

Perhaps the most challenging task for the group leader is helping group members do the hard work of tuning into the pain that resides beneath the off-putting behaviors of group members who suffer from Narcissistic Personality Disorder. Narcissists are people who, early in their lives, "decided" that an emotional investment in those responsible for their care was not worth making. With these important others, they had experienced more hate than love, more rejection than acceptance, and more indifference than compassion. They (unconsciously) withdrew whatever emotion they had placed in these important others and re-directed it to aspects of themselves. This emotional redistribution had two important consequences. First, it became vitally important to them *not* to be in touch with how desperately they needed emotional connection with other people. Second, instead of such connections, they now derived gratification and self-esteem from the workings of their minds, their material possessions, their physical appearance, or their worldly accomplishments. They lost touch with the emotional deprivation suffered early in life. Their need for admiration obscured their loneliness. Here are two examples.

William missed a group meeting and came late to the next one. As he entered the session, the group was involved in processing a heated interaction that had taken place between two members the week before. William kept interrupting the conversation to find out what had happened. The group did not interrupt its processing to bring William up to speed, something it most likely would have done if William had been a well-liked group member. In response to his fourth interruption, Helene said, "William, will you shut up." Without thinking, William retorted, "Helene, you bitch." After a brief silence, the group began criticizing William. I then directed a question to the group-as-a-whole, "How would members have felt if William had simply asked, 'Did you folks miss me last week?'" It was unanimous that if William had asked that question the group would have responded much differently. William looked sad and said that asking such a question would never occur to him. He didn't rely on other people for emotional sustenance. No wonder it was so difficult for others to detect his pain over the possibility that he was not missed.

Oliver, a veteran of group therapy, entered his first session in an ongoing group. Ten minutes into the group, Beverly entered late and the group took time to tell her what the group had been talking about. Like a Mack truck, Oliver interrupted the group's summary and announced that since Beverly was late, she should sit silently and catch up to the group's proceedings on her own. He also criticized the group for rewarding lateness with a summary. Not surprisingly, the group became very upset with Oliver who tried to justify his comments by citing his extensive experience as a group therapy patient.

Oliver's way of introducing himself to the group was not random. He had a history of many failed personal relationships, a major issue in his life that he had joined the group to work on. Within 15 minutes of being in the group he demonstrated a major difficulty: his compulsive need to show everyone how much he knew. Oliver's verbally assaultive behavior upset the group enough for 2 members to consider leaving the group. It took many months for the group to begin to learn about the emotional deprivation Oliver had suffered as a child growing up with psychologically damaged Holocaust survivor parents. The group's eventual caring for William helped him take an interest in other members' pain as well as to be vulnerable. These changes helped the group be able to empathize with his suffering.

There is one instance, alluded to in Chapter 19 (the very, very good patient), when it can be difficult to detect the pain of a patient who is *easy* to be with. Such a situation occurs with the patient who has an inordinate need to please and be "good"—often at his or her expense. With these patients it is not a matter of not wanting to acknowledge and deal with their pain; the problem is that they never make waves or indicate that they are in pain. Sally, a 35-year-old single woman with MS, was such a patient. It took a celebration of her birthday while she was a patient in an acute physical rehabilitation hospital to uncover her pain.

The rehabilitation team surrounded her bed and, after singing Happy Birthday, watched her cut the ice cream cake the nursing staff—who were very fond of her—had made for her. When invited to make a wish, Sally said, "Please make sure that the air-conditioner is not turned off." Snickers were evident among the amused, assembled staff. Someone asked her about her wish and she answered, "I have never had a birthday party before and I want to make sure that the cake doesn't melt." The deprivation embedded in her wish immediately changed the feeling in the room. Her pain was palpable.

Note

1 Feldman, M. (1997). Projective identification: The analyst's involvement. *Int J of Psychoanal*, (Pt 2): 227–241.

Index